Exercise Well with Autoimmunity

Exercise Well with Autoimmunity

Zoe Mckenzie

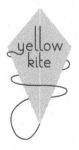

yellow
kite

First published in Great Britain in 2024 by Yellow Kite
An imprint of Hodder & Stoughton
An Hachette UK company

3

The information in this book is not intended to replace advice from a doctor or other health professional. If you have any concerns regarding your health or the suitability of the fitness plan for you, we recommend that you consult with your doctor before you embark on it. The author and publisher disclaim any liability directly or indirectly from the use of the material in this book by any person.

A CIP catalogue record for this title is available from the British Library

Trade Paperback ISBN 978 1 399 70852 4
ebook ISBN 978 1 399 70853 1
Audiobook ISBN 978 1 399 70854 8

Typeset in Sabon MT Std by Manipal Technologies Limited.

Printed and bound in Great Britain by Clays Ltd, Elcograf S.p.A.

Hodder & Stoughton policy is to use papers that are natural, renewable and recyclable products and made from wood grown in sustainable forests. The logging and manufacturing processes are expected to conform to the environmental regulations of the country of origin.

Yellow Kite
Hodder & Stoughton Ltd
Carmelite House
50 Victoria Embankment
London EC4Y 0DZ

www.yellowkitebooks.co.uk

Contents

Foreword

I am so pleased to be writing a foreword to Zoe Mckenzie's essential book on exercising well with an autoimmune condition. Movement is fundamental to living a healthy and happy life, however it can seem daunting when you are not feeling at your best. I know from personal experience that it can be challenging on so many fronts – you might be reluctant to get going with exercise, or have been told that you cannot, or perhaps you have tried it without the right guidance. This book provides everything you need to move forward into a regular form of exercise that works for you.

Zoe writes with compassion and understanding. Her exercise plans are supported by research, and will help you to move in your way, on your terms, for a better quality of life. Zoe draws upon her expertise as a physiotherapist, qualified Pilates instructor and personal trainer, as well as her deep personal understanding of what it is truly like to live with autoimmunity. Exercise has profound benefits on our physical, mental and emotional wellbeing and I have no doubt that implementing the suggestions found in the pages of this book will change your life for the better.

Emily Johnson
Author and Founder of Arthritis Foodie

Introduction: I get it

The most frequent feedback I get from my clients is that I 'get it'. Sometimes I wish I didn't get it quite so much. I wish that I haven't had to contend with so many medical conditions. But I have. And therefore, yes – I do get it.

I get the struggles of living with constant bone-deep fatigue. That heavy feeling of moving through concrete. I know that level of exhaustion, when even the walk to the kitchen for a glass of water feels impossible, no matter how thirsty I feel. I understand how even with the best understanding of pain psychology, pain can still be draining, all-encompassing and life-changing. I know how a sudden flare can put a stop to any movement, despite how motivated I may be.

I, too, experience the juggle of navigating an autoimmune condition while trying to live my life. It is ongoing, day after day, week after week, month after month. Living with ongoing health challenges is living, yes, and I'm grateful for that – but it is exhausting and draining. There is never a day off with regards to medication, supplements, medical admin, appointments, treatments and side effects. Just trying to manage my conditions as best I can takes up so much of my time and precious energy. I want to meet with friends. I want to work. I want to pull my weight, whether at home or in my relationships with friends and family. But chronic health conditions narrow that window of functioning, so narrowing the choices I can make. It can feel as though burning the candle at just one end is barely possible.

I have lower expectations of what is possible, compared to others of my age. And when my conditions flare, I have to lower them further still, until I'm down to the bare minimum. How then do you choose what to do (or what not to do) when you are already down to just the essential tasks? And how does exercise fit in with everything else?

At some point in the process, from when you first sought medical help for your symptoms to diagnosis and management, someone will have told you, 'You have to exercise'. I hope the language used around this was non-judgemental, compassionate and understanding of where you are in your health journey. I definitely hope it wasn't said in a way that was condescending, implying that you hadn't already thought of trying to exercise – or with blame, if your attempts had not been constructive. And I hope they didn't imply that nothing else can help you – that exercise is the only answer (it isn't; it's just one of many things that may support you). I hope, too, that they were able to refer you to a physiotherapist or group service to help you with how to exercise. That they didn't just leave you wondering how you are meant to exercise when you are exhausted and in pain all the time. And I hope that your experience of medical advice and exercise has been positive, but I know from my own encounters and from the stories of many others, that exercise advice can often be counterproductive.

Let's consider a typical scenario: you're coming to the end of a long-awaited check-up with your consultant. You have answered honestly and opened up to them about how hard everything is, and how much you are struggling. At this point, the word 'exercise' is mentioned. Maybe they quote the generic guidelines of 150 minutes a week. Maybe they just encourage exercise in general. Either way, it is meant well, but frequently lacking in practical support – and there is certainly no psychological support. Healthcare for chronic health conditions is under-resourced in the UK. In particular, younger people with chronic health conditions frequently face a lack of options. So if you are lucky enough to have a medical practitioner who does provide actual support with your journey with exercise, hold on to them and feed back to them how helpful this was.

The independent health industry can be hard to navigate. You have realised you are going to need some support with your movement journey. You start to google and suddenly, your screen is filled with options, all promising to help you progress and change your life. However, the more you read, the less sure you become. Personal trainers and fitness professionals vary widely in their training and experience. It is very possible that a personal trainer hasn't come across your condition before, and although this is not necessarily a reason not to work with them, it does depend on how they approach it.

You need a trainer who wants to learn *with* you: to read about your condition and, most importantly, listen to you. You will not be helped by someone who lacks experience or understanding of how health impacts your physiology and who gives you a plan set up for someone in good health, with no idea of how to adapt it to your body and how you feel. A trainer should be ready and willing to adapt any exercise session or programme to your level. Most of them love fitness and exercise, and therefore naturally struggle to comprehend what it feels like to live with fatigue and pain. Their programmes tend to get a person with chronic health conditions to do too much strength or cardiovascular work. And the consequences are far-reaching. Physically, this leads to a flare in symptoms; psychologically, it can cause depression and feelings of isolation and failure. The negative effects of inappropriate exercise are demotivating, and then most of us take the blame on ourselves: we are the failure and we are lazy. And we feel even more detached from the healthy world.

I am a physiotherapist. Training is standardised, quality checked, multi-layered and comprehensive. I believe physiotherapists are usually best placed to work with clients with autoimmune conditions. However, it does depend on what further training, courses and experience the individual therapist has undertaken and how their practice has developed. Some love hands-on work, whereas others take a completely exercise-based approach. Different methods – and therefore different physios – work for different clients. There are multiple other types of health practitioners, too: osteopaths, chiropractors, exercise physiologists, etc. The main thing when working with anyone is how that relationship feels to you. Trust your instincts, do your research, ask questions. Do they listen to you? Do they see you as the expert on your own body?

In addition to my physiotherapy and Pilates training, I completed a personal training course. Throughout the entire course there was only one mention of working with clients with disabilites. The lecturer said, 'If you have someone in a wheelchair, try to think of exercises they can do sitting down.' That was it! This is clearly grossly inadequate when it comes to chronic health conditions, but I am not here to criticise. Rather, what I hope to do is empower you, to help you believe in yourself. If you have had these experiences with exercise, it was not your fault. So be hopeful. Because there are ways you can reclaim movement for yourself.

Having said that, invisible illness does make things more challenging. If you turn up to your personal training session or Pilates class on crutches after an ankle sprain, they can instantly see and understand what you are dealing with and adapt your session accordingly. Walking in looking 'normal', but with invisible pain in various parts of your body is harder to understand and therefore it is harder to know how to adapt.

Then there is fatigue. Most people have encountered pain at one time or another, but fatigue can be more difficult to empathise with unless you – or someone you are close to – have experienced it. Everyone knows what tiredness feels like – we all get tired from work, from family life, from being busy. Maybe, someone of robust health has had a busy weekend of socialising, a rough night's sleep and an intense workout, but with a good, restorative night's sleep and perhaps a quieter schedule for a few days they can bounce back. The fatigue associated with chronic conditions is a different beast. It is the type of low energy where no amount of rest or sleep will help. We will go into fatigue more deeply in Chapter 11, but I think it is one of the most challenging symptoms when exercising, as we often feel ok in the moment, but then we are hit by complete physical and mental exhaustion, whether later that day or anywhere up to two or three days later. And trying to explain this to someone who thinks a warm-up is a jog and 100 burpees can be really challenging.

Pain management is another strand in chronic illness management. If you are fortunate, you may be placed in a condition- or age-specific group, which will hopefully give you more tailored advice. This can also be a great way to connect with others going through similar experiences, which, in itself, can be supportive and helpful. I was placed in a generic pain class where 90 per cent of the group were in their eighties with chronic back pain and therefore the advice was geared towards them. Sitting in an uncomfortable chair for longer than I could tolerate, being given vague, impractical advice was hardly inspiring, let alone helpful. Although not necessarily incorrect, the advice did not align with my goals, which were very different to those of my 'peers', which meant my rehab and exercise needs were vastly different, too. I found this demotivating and depressing and, sadly, many others I have come across have described a similar experience of these sessions. I do believe some of these services are improving and that with the right person organising and running the session they can be helpful and encouraging. Again, trust yourself: if you find the group you have been referred to useful, that's great! But if not, that's because it is not pitched at the right level for you. *It is not because you are doing it wrong.*

Another issue is the language and mindset around exercise. For example, if I see an article saying, 'Cure MS with exercise' I immediately dismiss it, as there is no current cure for MS, and the language used here adds pressure, implying you may not be doing enough or trying hard enough to get better if you are not exercising. However, if it says, 'Exercises to support your body' or, 'Movement to improve your function with MS', that is more appropriate. Living with any sort of chronic illness is really challenging and we don't need more stress or extra pressure from being simply told to exercise.

Many of my clients often believe they are lazy or unmotivated and blame themselves, so we spend time exploring where those thoughts have come from. Frequently, they say they don't like exercise, or don't want to do it because of how it has been framed previously or the type they have done before. I believe that no one is inherently lazy. You are not weak if you have tried but failed to make progress. You are blaming yourself, but it is not your fault.

You just haven't been shown *how* to exercise with your symptoms and your condition/s in a safe, effective way that will fit in with your lifestyle, and in a way you can actually enjoy.

Exercise *can* still be fun with autoimmune conditions – not a form of punishment or something you have to grit your teeth to get through. The general perception of exercise is that it has to be extreme in some way: pushing yourself to the max, sweating, red in the face. As if any other level of effort does not count. But this is completely incorrect. All movement counts – and understanding this can make a big difference in steering away from the all-or-nothing mindset that often dominates the exercise arena. The main thing is to find out the real reason why someone wants to exercise and to focus on building a consistent routine that suits them.

I hate anything that's preachy, bossy or implies that there is a right or wrong way to exercise. It's about finding what works with you and your body. This book, therefore, will give you all the tips and tricks I have picked up from my experiences as a physiotherapist, Pilates instructor and personal trainer living and moving with multiple chronic illnesses. I want to do this with kindness to you and your body, so that introducing more movement into your life is positive for you, both physically and emotionally.

So here is my pledge to you:
- I will not preach or boss you around or add any pressure to exercise; this is important to me – this is a guide for when you want to exercise, to make it easier and more accessible.
- I will not dictate that there is a right or wrong way to exercise; we are all individuals, with different conditions (or combinations of conditions), pain thresholds, lifestyles and goals.

- I will not give advice around diet or weight management. I am not qualified to give out tailored nutrition guidance, nor would I want to. Nutrition is highly complex and varies alongside medication, supplements and dietary needs. Physical activity can have a role in weight management, but so many other factors also need to be addressed. In no way do I want to encourage unhealthy methods for losing weight or for promoting any kind of shame or guilt surrounding exercise and body size. All bodies are welcome here.
- I will not insist that you try movement if exercise is not an option for you right now. Perhaps you are coping with medical challenges or you simply do not have the headspace to add this to your toolbox right now. Nobody needs any more 'shoulds', pressure or stress in their life. Exercise is here for you whenever you feel ready to choose to move your body.

Beginning with my own journey, I will take you through the benefits of exercises to how to set yourself up with a consistent exercise routine that works for you. I will then guide you through strength exercises, with options in different positions, and mobility movements. I will give you the tools to be able to adapt movement to your fluctuating symptoms and talk through some of the challenges we face with our mindsets and movement.

I hope my guiding principles and experience from working with a wide range of clients all over the world will help you, whenever the time is right for you, to find your foundations and direction with movement to support you in living your life in the best way possible for you.

1

My journey
with movement

I have always loved exercise. Although I probably didn't grow up thinking of it as exercise – it was just having fun, being part of a team or going on adventures. I think having an older brother spurred me on, too, giving me the mentality of 'whatever he can do, I can do' from a young age. Not surprising, then, that my first swimming experience involved me launching myself off the side of the pool independently. I had on one of those swimming costumes with the floats around the middle, which meant I had to keep my head up myself (unlike with traditional armbands), and my mum says she spent the next twenty minutes trying to help me, but whenever she touched me, I'd push her away, determined to do what my brother, Rory, was doing. He didn't need Mum's help, so neither would I.

I started ballet when I was very young and loved it, despite my teacher calling me 'banana legs'. I picked up jazz, modern and tap and used to dance my way around life with dreams of being a ballerina. I loved our yearly dance shows and, as I grew older, I took part in competitions, both locally and in London. I even won the ballet cup – probably my favourite award to date. Alongside dancing, after my dramatic introduction to the water, I continued to swim and began competing for our local team – again, both locally and for our county. My banana legs that weren't so useful in ballet were very helpful with breaststroke, as my tight adductor muscles (inner thighs) and great range of hip movement meant my kick was strong and I often beat swimmers twice my size.

At school, I took part in most of the sports on offer. Other than anything requiring hand–eye co-ordination, that is – even in senior school, I never made it past the baby net in tennis, and I have yet to return a volley; in hockey I would forever be running, thinking I had the ball pressed to my hockey stick, only to look back and realise the game was playing out behind me, as I had successfully missed the ball. In hindsight, my proprioception, spatial awareness and posture were all signs that something was going on for me. At the time, of course, I just thought I was useless at certain things.

Looking through my old school notebooks recently, I came across something I wrote when I was just seven years old: 'My favourite time of the day is playtime, although my legs get really tired from running'. Reading that my younger self experienced fatigue made me realise how long I have lived with a body that is different to others'.

Nevertheless, despite always being a little different, I loved sport and moving my body. I wasn't naturally competitive, and my parents were definitely not pushy – they were more surprised when I did well, rather than expecting it or putting pressure on me. I loved the feeling of moving my body, of being part of something. I made such good friends both swimming and dancing and loved being part of a team, both for the sports and performance. Exercise back then wasn't about any of things that society or the medical profession lecture us on today. It wasn't about losing weight or gaining muscle strength. It was about enjoyment, friendships and challenging yourself. I hold on to these joys as I navigate exercise as an adult.

For the first thirteen years of my life, I was very active. Then came my first injury, on the netball pitch. I like to imagine that it happened as I landed from scoring the crucial goal that led to us winning the match. However, I have no recollection as to whether the ball went into the net or not, or if we won or lost. I just remember jumping up and then landing and knowing something wasn't right. I had no prior experience of injury, so I had no expectation of the pain or how long it should take to improve. I am grateful now that I was so ignorant, as this small injury took over five years to heal. My physiotherapy rehab started at this time – the classic exercise band around the ankle and hours and hours doing tiny, repetitive movements. I was keen to get back to dancing and swimming, plus all my sports in general at school, so I persevered, balancing on wobble boards and jumping on mini trampolines.

A few months later, I started to swim again, just doing arm drills and not using my legs – but I soon dislocated my shoulder. I then added shoulder rehab to my exercises, with more exercise bands, gentle strength work and lots of sticker charts to keep me motivated. Another few months later, pain was spreading into all my joints, which didn't make sense at the time. My injuries were in my ankle and shoulder, so why was the pain affecting other areas? And I was struggling to sleep and function, too.

It was becoming clear that more was going on here, and my GP referred me to a paediatrician. They ran some blood tests and declared that as I didn't have juvenile arthritis, they had no idea what was wrong. I was then passed around to several local doctors, including a rheumatologist who could not see why I was deteriorating and kept asking me if I was being bullied.

Meanwhile, I kept up with my exercises, and my physiotherapists were always kind and understanding, but it was an awful time. In the end, my mum insisted on a referral for specialist help. I was sent to Great Ormond Street Hospital (GOSH) and was immediately diagnosed with Ehlers-Danlos syndrome (EDS). At GOSH, they understood the negative cycle on pain and injury that I was in, and it was so good, finally, to be believed and understood. EDS is a group of disorders caused by genetic changes that affect connective tissue and how the genes provide instructions for making collagen and other proteins. This influences how the body functions, due to the soft tissues being structured differently, causing joint hypermobility, while also impacting skin elasticity, as well as bladder and bowel function, among other things.

As a teenager, I presented with musculoskeletal issues, chronic pain and fatigue. By the time I was able to access treatment, I had been in a wheelchair for six months, unable to walk more than a few metres, and I would only do stairs once a day to flop into bed, where I would lie awake all night with insomnia.

Through intensive rehab at GOSH I was taught how to walk again, to regain a normal gait (pattern of movement/walking) and slowly and steadily build up my strength and stamina. I was taught to push through the pain, that the pain wasn't useful or helpful to me and that I was the only person who could help myself. I was the one who had to do my exercises every single day or I would end up back in my wheelchair.

I took all this completely to heart, perhaps being a little too hard on myself, but I was terrified of taking a backward step and so desperately wanted to get better. I was mid-teens by this point – grumpy, a little withdrawn, trying to grow up and be a normal teenager but also having to be diligent with my exercise programme. Some days, it would feel so hard – mentally, just to get myself on the mat in the first place and physically, because my limbs felt as if they were made of lead. Tears would stream down my face as I counted out thirty reps of everything, over and over again, to keep myself strong.

I kept up my exercises through the rest of my school years, through college and up to university, where I wanted to study to be a physiotherapist, having seen the difference they can make. I dropped my 'rehab' style of exercises and was finding more 'normal' ways to move my body again through going to the gym, yoga, Pilates. I also started to run – more and more. I knew I had to keep myself strong, so despite the usual stresses of studying, I always made sure to prioritise movement. On reflection, I think I pushed myself too hard. I was motivated to keep going through fear of regressing and knowing that it was up to me to manage my condition.

It started to feel like my body was falling apart bit by bit as I got older – not just my joints now, but living with chronic migraine, and the onset of digestive problems and bladder dysfunction too. I used movement as a coping tool. It gave me a fleeting sense of power over a body that felt very much out of my control. By my final year of university, I was running up to twice a day and doing core and strengthening work. I graduated with a first. However, I was well and truly exhausted, and after university, I knew I needed time out to support my body and mind.

After some time at home to recover, I decided to accept a physiotherapy job in Sydney, Australia. It did feel slightly mad, considering my health issues, but my determination to not let my health stop me spurred me on. Once there, I was more active than ever. Partly because everyone there is outside and exercising and partly because I was broke, and without a car, I preferred walking to getting slow, busy buses.

I was working as a physiotherapist in elderly care, which was physically demanding, as well as running exercise groups and giving up to thirty hands-on treatments a day. I would then run most nights after work, as I loved the freedom it gave me. It felt like flying, but I think that was just the beautiful scenery and my motivating playlist (I think most people could walk faster than I ran) – and no matter how tough the first twenty minutes were, or how awful I felt on my way up the hill to home, I was so grateful to be running again after years of not being able to.

One thing I neglected was my strength regime. Since moving to Sydney and being so active, I'd told myself I didn't need it any more. I sustained a few smaller injuries, which I stupidly ignored, until back pain started, forcing me to listen. I wasn't new to pain, but this completely floored me. I was on the other side of the world from my family and usual physiotherapist. I had rent to pay and my work visa required me to work thirty-eight hours a week. At the time, my focus was on my physical symptoms but, on reflection, there were huge psychological, emotional and money stresses, too. My back injury came with an increase in fatigue levels. I was stuck in that awful cycle of pain, both in my back and referring down my left leg, causing sleeplessness at night, and days spent completely exhausted. It was as if my whole nervous system was vibrating and wired incorrectly. And so, for the hundredth time in my life, I started rehab.

I realised, once again, that I would have to be the one to help myself. I started the two things that had supported my body time and time again and got me strong again: swimming and Pilates. I began with walking up and down the pool, then managing to swim two lengths, then four, then six, until I was swimming over a kilometre at a time. I spent the first few Pilates sessions missing out quite a lot of the class or adapting it, but I built up, until I was doing all the advanced work. And I kept walking, gradually increasing what I could manage. Some days I overdid it, and at night the pain would flare, while other times it would be tolerable, and I'd build up again. I had to have more rests, and my energy levels didn't go back to where they were before, but I was strong enough to return to work. Movement had helped me back on my feet again.

After this, I knew I had to keep up the movement that suited me best. I loved running for my mental health, but my physical health needed more supportive strategies. It was like I had spent the first eight months of my life in Sydney trying to run away from my health issues – literally. So I continued to swim and do Pilates; I also joined a gym and went back to strength training, determined to get myself as strong as possible.

Adding in these supportive exercise strategies helped and I became the strongest I had ever been since my EDS diagnosis. I then moved to my dream job and was teaching Pilates, alongside physiotherapy work, which I loved, but the hours were long and tough. I was doing forty plus hours a week, and I knew in my gut it wasn't sustainable. And I was right.

A lingering cold for a couple of months turned into me becoming acutely unwell. I had severe right-sided abdominal pain, flu-like symptoms, fevers, sweats (especially at night) and couldn't even stand upright. Initially, it was thought that I had appendicitis, but after removing a healthy appendix and my subsequent failure to recover, I was told I had 'mesenteric adenitis' (a fancy way of saying I had enlarged lymph nodes, showing my stomach was inflamed and struggling).

As always, I took it on myself to recover from my latest weird health thing, thinking it was another episode that I would handle. I started the rehab process again, beginning with very gentle Pilates. I managed to recuperate from the surgery, but as the weeks turned into months, it became harder and harder to exercise and I was still unable to return to work. My fatigue worsened, I had fevers and sharp, stabbing pains, I was covered in a rash, had ongoing flu-like symptoms and could barely eat, due to constant nausea and vomiting multiple times a day. I underwent what felt like a million blood tests and scans, ruling out various conditions, until, eventually, I was diagnosed with systemic lupus erythematosus (SLE, or lupus, for short – an autoimmune disease in which the immune system attacks its own tissues, causing widespread inflammation and tissue damage in the affected areas). I started my love/hate relationship with steroids – love because they made me feel so much better, hate because of the wild side effects and hideous weaning off. I also had to take immunosuppressants and hydroxychloroquine (an anti-malarial drug that works to decrease the activity of the immune system, so helping treat rheumatic conditions).

The more I learned and read about lupus, the more I realised that my usual approach of 'pushing through' wouldn't work this time, since my body was in a highly reactive state, and my immune system was in overdrive.

Still, I continued to exercise in ways I could, with strength training Pilates-style workouts, but they were more intermittent than before and often shorter. I started to adapt my training to find a balance that suited me, and to relearn how my body responded to exercise. In so doing, I realised the biggest thing I was changing was not so much *how* I was exercising, but my mindset around movement. I was learning to listen to my body, lying on my mat, adapting my exercise plan depending on my health that day. Following my lupus diagnosis, I was officially diagnosed with PoTS (postural orthostatic tachycardia syndrome), a condition affecting the autonomic nervous system which controls your heart rate and blood pressure, although it was thought I had lived with it for some time. My bladder was always temperamental, but my function deteriorated when I was sick with lupus, I needed a supra pubic catheter placed, and my migraine attacks worsened too. I had to keep adjusting and figuring out how to support my body because of the constant medical tests, procedures and surgeries, along with ever changing medication and fluctuating symptoms.

Now, seventeen years after my initial injury, I know my body so well. I know what I can manage with my symptoms, I can tune in and recognise when it needs rest and when it needs movement. I know which pains need medical attention and which are telling me to slow down and calm my nervous system. I feel I have found a balance, where movement continues to bring me joy and prevent further injury, and I work *with* my body, rather than pushing it all the time.

All this has brought me to where I am today. In many ways I have become the physiotherapist I needed myself, except that I am now able to help others around the world with my personal insight into how chronic illness really feels. I don't think I could ever say I am glad to have lupus, but that diagnosis did lead me to where I am professionally, and I love what I get to do now (including writing this book!).

The benefits of exercising with autoimmune conditions

Most of us know that moving our bodies is good for us. Routine physical activity has been shown to:

- improve muscular and cardiorespiratory fitness
- improve bone health
- improve cardiometabolic health (the health of your heart, blood and blood vessels)
- help manage body composition
- improve mental health, including reducing symptoms of anxiety and depression
- improve sleep quality
- prevent several chronic conditions, such as cardiovascular disease, diabetes, cancer, hypertension, obesity and osteoporosis
- improve autonomic tone (supporting the balance of the nervous system)
- reduce chronic inflammation
- reduce the risk of premature death.

I hope that at some point during your health journey so far, someone has mentioned the benefits of exercising with your condition. I also hope that you haven't experienced the other extreme, where your health concerns have been dismissed with comments such as, 'If you lost weight or tried exercise, you would be ok'. As far as I am concerned, anyone who promises that exercise is a cure should be politely ignored. I adopt a happy-medium approach, whereby exercise is helpful and an important strategy in my toolbox for managing my conditions, but there should be no blame or feelings of guilt if you don't dramatically improve or cannot do as much as others with the same condition.

Understanding the place of exercise within the overall management of your condition is important. Just as medication, nutrition and supplements all play a part, so does exercise. Research is promising in showing that exercise has an anti-inflammatory effect, can prevent future complications or other health conditions from developing and can help with pain, fatigue and mental health when implemented in the right way. It can help you feel more in control of your body and to reconnect with yourself after being unwell.

Exercise and autoimmune conditions

There are thought to be over eighty different types of autoimmune conditions with many more suspected to be autoimmune, too. Our immune systems usually protect our bodies, but with an autoimmune condition they mistake healthy tissues for foreign, attacking them as a result. Where they attack and the impact this has will vary, manifesting in different types of autoimmune conditions. Below is a breakdown of some of the most common ones, along with the research on exercising with them.

Rheumatoid arthritis (RA)

RA is a chronic, systemic autoimmune disease impacting joint health, leading to pain, inflammation, fatigue and decreased muscle mass (known as rheumatoid cachexia). More than 80 per cent of RA patients are physically inactive, which can become a vicious cycle with both general health and disease progression. Exercise has been shown to help reverse cachexia and improve function without exacerbating the disease. It also helps to reduce the risk of cardiovascular disease, improve bone density and general health outcomes. Intensive exercise does not increase the damage to the large joints, unless considerable baseline damage is already seen in scans prior to starting.

Multiple sclerosis (MS)

MS affects the central nervous system, due to damage to the protective sheath (myelin) around the nerve fibres in the brain and spinal cord. This can cause lesions in the nervous system and affects how messages are sent around the body, leading to muscle spasms, weakness, loss of co-ordination and balance, fatigue, neural symptoms such as pins and needles, pain, continence issues, cognitive decline and vertigo or dizziness. Many patients avoid physical activity due to fear of worsening symptoms or not knowing how best to exercise with their condition. However, research shows that exercise can help to reduce deconditioning and improve patients' ability to function. Exercise can help manage physical and mental symptoms without triggering any flares of the condition or a relapse. Aerobic training with low to moderate intensity can improve fatigue, while strength training can help with functional movements like walking and stairs, and balance retraining can help prevent falls and further injuries. Flexibility exercises can also help to manage spasticity (tightening or stiffening of muscles) and prevent future complications like contractions (when a limb becomes fixed in one position).

Lupus

Lupus is a chronic inflammatory disease with a wide range of clinical presentations due to its effect on multiple organ systems. There are four main types of lupus: neonatal, discoid, drug-induced and systemic lupus erythematosus (SLE). Lupus can present with fever, fatigue and weight loss, as well as rashes, mouth ulcers/sores, painful and/or stiff joints, with or without swelling and muscle pain. It can affect the respiratory, cardiovascular, gastrointestinal, renal and haematological systems, as well as the central nervous system.

In general, exercise has been shown to improve many of the musculoskeletal symptoms in lupus. It has been shown to be safe and there is no evidence of harm or increased disease activity following exercise. Upper-limb exercises have shown significant improvement for hand function, pain, daily activity and overall quality of life. Many studies have found that SLE patients have lower cardiovascular capacity than healthy people and lower physical fitness, muscle strength and functional capacity, all of which can be improved with routine exercise. There is some research that exercise can improve fatigue levels.

Inflammatory bowel disease

IBD is a group of autoimmune disorders involving chronic inflammation in the digestive tract. This includes ulcerative colitis (inflammation and ulcers along the lining of the colon and rectum) and Crohn's disease (inflammation of any part of the gastrointestinal tract, from the mouth to the rectum). Symptoms can include diarrhoea, rectal bleeding, abdominal pain, fatigue and joint pain.

Research shows that there is no danger of disease or symptom exacerbation with mild to moderate exercise and it may even help to reduce the risk of constipation, diverticular disease and colorectal cancer. Along with the usual benefits of exercise, it can also help to increase bone mineral density (BMD), which is especially important, as IBD patients often have low BMD. The anti-inflammatory properties of exercise may also be helpful in managing the condition. There is limited research on specific details about type, intensity and frequency, but overall, exercise has been shown to help quality of life for patients living with IBD.

Type 1 diabetes mellitus

Diabetes is a chronic condition, where the body does not make enough insulin or cannot use it effectively to regulate the glucose (sugar) released when eating carbohydrates. Normally, insulin opens the channels to let glucose move from the bloodstream into the body's cells to be used as energy. However, with type 1 diabetes, which is an autoimmune condition, the body attacks itself, preventing the pancreas from producing insulin. Symptoms include increased thirst, passing more urine, feeling tired and lethargic, slow healing of wounds and skin infections, nausea and vomiting, weight loss and mood swings.

Physical exercise is key in the management of diabetes due to the general cardiovascular health benefits which are important in preventing future complications. Regular exercise improves overall health outcomes, including helping with blood-sugar levels. There are very few risks to exercising with diabetes; however, exercise should be avoided when blood-sugar values are excessively high or low. Many patients avoid or fear exercise due to worries about managing blood-glucose levels, but increasing options for glucose-monitoring technology and improved education from medical teams have helped more patients to exercise regularly. The impact of exercise on an individual's blood-sugar levels varies, depending on the type, intensity and duration of the activity, and can be balanced by adjusting the insulin dose, as well as with carbohydrate and fluid intake. Resistance (strength) exercises tend to lead to a much smaller drop in blood sugars during the activity than aerobic movement, and require less carbohydrate supplementation. Exercising can lead to nocturnal hypoglycaemia (low blood sugar overnight) which needs to be monitored, especially for anyone who is relatively new to movement or making big changes to their activity plan.

Connecting with your body

Something that research doesn't pick up on is how having a long-term health condition can alter the way you feel about your body. When I was struggling with new symptoms, I felt disconnected from my body, as I didn't understand what was going on with it. It felt foreign and different, and I no longer felt like an expert in it. When I was diagnosed, I felt betrayed by my body. How could it have yet another thing wrong with it? I didn't know how to manage this new condition, how my body would respond, whether I would get better.

When we are in pain, our brains try to block it out, pretend it's not there. And although in the short term, blocking everything out can feel helpful in trying to survive, living in such a disconnected way is not constructive in the long term. A common theme throughout this book is learning to listen to your body and work *with* it, as a team, and that's pretty hard to do if you are constantly trying to ignore it. But movement can help you to reconnect. It gives you the time and space in your day to check in with your body and notice how things feel – to start listening to it again.

Exercise helped me to rebuild trust in my body. At a time when I was unable to work, socialise or function, gradually seeing improvements in my strength or ability to walk helped me to feel like I was accomplishing something. It boosted my self-efficacy, giving me a sense of being in control of my health. I have also seen the positive impact of exercise on others' relationships with their bodies – and I know it can do the same for you, too.

3

Goals and motivation

There are two main types of motivation: extrinsic and intrinsic. Extrinsic motivation can be described as behaviour driven by external rewards or punishments – these may be tangible, like playing tennis to win a trophy. Or a more conceptual extrinsic motivator would be social standing or shame – for example, exercising so your doctor does not tell you off for being inactive. Frequently, someone, somewhere is telling you that you should exercise, and this can lead to feelings of guilt or failure if you struggle to build a consistent routine. Most of us tend to respond well when we are being held accountable by someone else (say, through regular sessions with a trainer or going to the gym with a friend), but if we rely purely on someone else to motivate us, our whole exercise routine can falter if any aspect of this changes (say, if your trainer cancels a session or your friend's schedule doesn't work with yours).

Motivation can also come from an intrinsic place – from goals you want to achieve for yourself (for example, wanting to manage to climb the stairs pain free, or doing an activity just because you enjoy it). Researchers have come up with the four Cs of intrinsic motivation: challenge, curiosity, control and context. The challenge aspect can help you to feel worthy or self-accomplished if you achieve it. Curiosity drives you to learn something new and improve some aspect of yourself without external reward. You might be motivated to do something in order to feel a sense of control over your environment. And context is about having the relevant skills to help solve problems.

There is no right or wrong way to motivate yourself. Equally, your motivation does not have to come solely from an intrinsic or extrinsic place but can be a combination of the two – for example, wanting to run a marathon for the medal and social approbation, as well as for the sense of achievement from the challenge. I believe the best way to motivate yourself is to find a reason – or reasons – that are meaningful to you. Why do you want to add in more physical activity?

Understanding why you are going to make yourself move is important for anyone, but especially when you are living with pain and fatigue. I use the following scenario, inspired by my own experience: imagine you have flopped on to the sofa. You feel tired and your pain levels are high. But you still need to find some energy to cook dinner and get ready for bed. What is going to motivate you in that moment to get from the sofa to your mat? It may be a seemingly small and very specific reason or it may be a more general internally held belief. But either way, it has to be powerful – powerful enough to help you navigate a path through the physical and mental barriers to exercise you have acquired (more on this in the next chapter).

If you find yourself saying, 'It will be good for me' or, 'My doctor wants me to exercise more' or, 'I want to feel stronger', I want you to dig deeper behind those thoughts. Ask yourself *why* will it be good for you? *Why* do you want to do what your doctor said? *Why* do you want to feel stronger? What would doing these things mean to you or bring to your life? Be your own therapist – keep digging, until you get to the underlying reason why you want to start adding in movement. The following table will help you with this process – use it to get to the bottom of your personal 'why'.

I want to feel stronger.

Why?

Because being strong helps me to be able
to sit up for longer or walk for longer.

But why do you need that?

Sitting up enables me to be at my desk to
work and walking helps with leaving the house
and spending time with my family.

Why is that important to you?

My work is meaningful to me – I love time
with my clients, and I love small adventures with
my family.

Why?

I want to be the strongest I can be to enable
me to work, to function and live a happy life.

Once you have completed this process, write your 'why' on a sticky note and stick it on a mirror or your desk, make it your phone background or write it in your diary. Surround yourself with your motivation in this way, repeating to yourself why you want to move. Let it be your mantra – how exercise is going to open up opportunities and possibilities for you to live your life in the way that is most meaningful to you. This is what *I* come back to, time and time again, when I am tired and in pain and I need that motivation to get on my mat.

Building a habit

> A habit is a settled or regular tendency or practice, especially one that is hard to give up.
>
> *Oxford English Dictionary*

So you've identified your motivation. Perhaps you are geared up to start a new exercise programme or try a new class. Maybe you print out a calendar to track the days and you get everything you need, so you're ready to start. Day 1: you feel great, you are enthusiastic, excited, even! Day 2: you feel ok; perhaps somewhat less excited, maybe a little sore from day 1. Day 3: this feels more of a drag, and then maybe you miss days 4 and 5, as you are busy and can't bring yourself to catch up. And before you know it, you have the stopped the whole thing and gone back to doing nothing.

Motivation alone isn't enough to get you to keep to a regular routine of movement – or anything, for that matter. It helps you to start, but a habit is what helps you to continue. Habits help you to integrate a new activity into your routine and to keep that pattern going. Routine helps you to do 'the thing', without putting too much thought into it, and then to keep doing it – because that, in turn, is a motivator.

Take brushing your teeth, for example. When you were younger, you probably went through a stage of not enjoying brushing your teeth, as you did not fully appreciate why it was necessary and there didn't appear to be any real short-term benefit. Your parents might have tried to explain that the dentist would tell you off if you didn't brush your teeth, or maybe the dentist themselves used scare tactics, telling you your teeth would fall out if you didn't brush them (both examples of extrinsic fear-based motivation). Or maybe you were tempted by some disgusting fruit-flavoured highly coloured toothpaste (bribery) or you had a sticker chart to help you track your progress to help with your motivation and habit building. Whatever the motivation, though, over time, brushing your teeth became a habit – something you do twice a day for two minutes, without thinking too much about it – and you grew to understand the associated benefits (and risks of doing not doing it). You now no longer have to plan it into your day, you don't have to leave notes as reminders or need a sticker chart (although no shame if you do – I still love a sticker chart and regularly use them, both for myself and for clients when building new habits).

Making movement a habit is much the same. If you can get into a routine of adding it into your daily life, it takes far less effort and energy to remember to do so. Building the habit in the first place is the hard part, and there are approximately a hundred books out there telling you how best to do it. I know – because I have read so many of them! But James Clear's *Atomic Habits* (see Resources, p. 235) resonated the most with me and my experience of trying to build habits alongside chronic illness. He sets out a four-step model, comprising cue, craving, response and reward. Once your cue (the trigger to initiate the behaviour) and craving (the motivational drive behind it) are aligned, it's time to focus on your response (the habit you will implement), so that you set yourself up for success – aka your reward – when integrating your exercise habit.

Now, let's start with frequency and duration. Aiming to do something every day from the get-go – walking, for example – might be quite challenging, so you may want to start by aiming for three days a week. This helps to set you up for success, then you can gradually build up to however many days a week you can manage, depending on how it goes and how you feel. When it comes to duration, you may want to walk for thirty minutes but, again, that might not be achievable straight away, so instead consider starting with a five-minute walk, then build up the time to thirty minutes as you become more consistent and the habit becomes a part of your routine. If you do manage more days than planned or longer than intended, that's a bonus – extra stickers on the chart! – and it helps to boost your confidence and self-efficacy.

Once you have built a consistent, safe and achievable routine, my advice is to stick rigidly to it (as far as possible, given your chronic condition) to help set up the habit. Some theories suggest it takes twenty-one days for a habit to stick, but in reality, it can take anywhere from two to eight months, depending on the individual and the behaviour they are trying to change. So if you don't manage to achieve what you set out for the week, try not to be hard on yourself. It is hard to integrate something new; it takes a bit of trial and error. Have a think about what's prevented you from achieving your goal and make a new plan for the next week. It has been found that missing a day or a session does not impact the formation of the habit – the main thing is trying to get back into it when you can. I recommend aiming for no more than two rest days in a row, and then on the third day doing something – anything – even if you just do one exercise on that third day. Because the more days you take off in a row, the harder it is to get back into the swing of things. However, if you do miss more than two days, that's ok, too. It's about continuing with exercise as soon as you are able. Don't let missing sessions derail the habit you are trying to create – keep trying.

Another useful tool is 'habit stacking', which is when you stack your new habit with something you already do without any thought. For example, I always make my morning coffee at 10am, then I will do my exercise after my coffee. Or I will do my mobility exercises after I brush my teeth and before bed. This way you are linking your habit to a task that is already automatic, which helps you to remember it. Context can also be helpful to initiate a behaviour, especially for exercising at home. You might leave your mat out at home, for example, then when you see it, you will remember to do your exercises. I find that making my exercise equipment accessible helps because it is a reminder to move my body, and also means that less energy is required to get everything ready. When I first was diagnosed with lupus and was unable to work, I used to exercise every time I watched *Love Island* – to this day, the theme music reminds me of lying down on my mat and starting!

Goals

Goal setting can be problematic with chronic illness because of the fluctuations in health and function on any given day. You may have come across SMART goals – specific, measurable, achievable, realistic and timely. This approach to goal setting encourages a focus on something useful and meaningful. Thinking and planning out the practicable steps needed can lead to a better chance of success in achieving your goal.

However, recent research has shown that other goal-setting techniques can be just as beneficial. Non-specific, open goals have resulted in more success and improved sustainability, so instead of 'I want to walk 5km in twenty minutes', you could say, 'I want to see how far I can walk in twenty minutes'. These type of open-ended goals have been shown to be more motivating than ones that could either be too easy or, conversely, too daunting, adding an element of enjoyment and a challenge. It has also been shown that we respond positively to challenges, so sometimes, too realistic a goal doesn't drive us to complete it.

I adapt goal setting when working with clients, depending on the challenges and situations they face as individuals. I like to set SMAR goals, losing the T, i.e. the time pressure. This is because chronic health conditions add a level of jeopardy that is not within our control. We can be on track with reaching a goal, then, out of nowhere, we are hit with a flare or an infection or a hospital procedure. At best, life can feel like a game of snakes and ladders, but when living with chronic illness the game changes: fewer ladders, more snakes and longer ones, threatening to take us back down the board, again and again. And even though we know these setbacks are outside of our control, we can feel at fault, taking on the failure of missing the deadline for the goal we had hoped to achieve. So removing that time pressure helps us to stay compassionate to ourselves and our bodies when challenged with setbacks due to ill health and keeps our focus on taking that next step forward or finding those ladders.

Goals created with a healthy intention, flexibility and compassion can be a helpful addition to identifying your 'why' and working on creating a habit for movement. However, it is neither essential nor always helpful to set goals. For some people, setting goals and then failing to reach them can be demotivating and lead to feeling that trying to exercise is pointless. For some, the nature of their condition is that things will deteriorate over time, and therefore it is about working from the place they are at now, rather than focusing on the future. For others, their health is precarious, and an event such as an infection can have a knock-on effect on something else, which then makes something else worse in turn. Again, if this is a current pattern, focusing on supporting your body in the moment is good enough.

With all this in mind, the next part is optional. If you currently feel that having a goal would not be helpful, then move on to the next chapter. If, however, you feel that it will help to give you a clear direction, read on.

Goal setting in practice

The following are examples of goal setting in relation to an underlying 'why':

Client 1

Client 1 has fibromyalgia with chronic migraine. She is currently unable to do any cooking – something she used to love doing and was a very important part of her life. She wants to share this role with her husband, but every time she tries to be in the kitchen, it leads to a flare and, as a result, she now associates it with pain and fears being in there.

Why: to be able to cook again with her husband and to host her friends for dinner, as it brings her joy.

Goals:

- To be able to stand for up to ten minutes at a time in the kitchen
- To build upper-body strength to help with tasks like chopping, mixing and carrying
- To build up confidence in her ability to cook without triggering a pain flare

Action plan:

- To add in a strength programme to help support upper body for cooking tasks and to help lower body feel stronger for standing
- To start with cooking a small simple dish she feels familiar with and can do within ten minutes
- To sit down for all tasks where it is safe to do so – for example, chopping
- To take ten-minute rest breaks throughout cooking stages – say, after three minutes of chopping vegetables or after putting something in the oven
- To ask for assistance from her husband when needed, to reduce the load and share the task

Client 2

Client 2 has rheumatoid arthritis and is not currently stable as they are in between medications. They want to stay as active as possible, despite pain levels being high and fatigue worse than usual. They also are still trying to work and socialise and juggle everything, so not much is left over in their energy tank for exercise.

Why: to enjoy movement again and be able to support joints as best they can.

Goals:
- To try to walk once a week for ten minutes at a minimum
- To try to do mobility exercises on Monday mornings before work
- To have a consistent routine, even with high pain levels

Action plan:
- To set up a short mobility programme that fits into the time available before work
- To plan out the week by looking at overall activity levels and decide which day would be best for adding in the ten-minute walk
- To use the toolbox of management techniques to help calm the nervous system to aid with pain and relaxation

You can see from these two examples how goals can vary, depending on what is going on for the individual and what matters to them. For some clients, we keep goals more general – for example, to add in movement three times a week. Then, once that has become a sustainable habit, we might start to narrow it down, maybe focusing on a health- or skill-related goal.

Health-related goals are based on the components of physical fitness, such as body composition, muscle endurance and strength, cardiovascular endurance and flexibility. This is often where we start when we reintroduce exercise. Skill-related goals are more performance related, such as improving balance, co-ordination, agility, speed, power and reaction time. These types of goals become more relevant when you have a strong baseline and can start to reintroduce specific exercise or sport, like getting back to tennis or rock climbing.

For other clients we set 'minimum goals'; as the name suggests, these are the bare minimum they want to try to achieve – for example, one strength session a week. This can sometimes feel more achievable, and anything else on top of this is a bonus, especially when everything feels overwhelming, or their health feels unsteady. This also links back to helping set people up for success with a sustainable habit. Lastly, for some clients, we just focus on their why and do not worry about goals.

So the bottom line when it comes to goal setting is that it all depends on you as an individual and how you prefer to think and motivate yourself.

Goal workbook

The following questions may be helpful in identifying your 'why', assessing your goals and planning how to implement them.

Why do I want to exercise?

How do I want to feel through exercise?

If someone waved a magic wand and I could do any physical activity again, what would I choose?

What do I think is stopping me from being able to do this?

Is there a way I can modify this or break the activity down?

Three habits I want to introduce to help me work towards my why or my goal:

4

Barriers to exercising

According to the World Health Organization (WHO), more than a quarter of the world's adult population (1.4 billion) are insufficiently active. Everyone has reasons why they struggle to hit those target physical-activity goals per week, whether that's a lack of financial resources, lack of time, lack of support or guidance and more. I call these barriers to exercising, and they are all valid, as well as varying between individuals.

Exercising with a chronic illness adds even more barriers – navigating symptoms, medication, hospital trips or appointments, changes in your body that feel out of your control and not being able to access the right support to help you as an individual to exercise. And the latter is so important, as too much movement or exercising in a way that doesn't suit your body can lead to negative consequences, making it even harder to encourage yourself to exercise again.

The hardest part of exercising according to most of my clients is consistency. Everyone can do something once – the challenge is repeating it, week in, week out, adapting it to what your body can do. And when your body is fluctuating, whether with flares or changes to medication, for example, it's even harder.

It is not your fault if movement is a struggle. And it is ok if some weeks exercise is less of a priority or does not happen in the way you planned. It is all right if it takes a while before you can build up that consistency; as discussed in the previous chapter with your why and your goals, habits take a while to build. You shouldn't be hard on yourself, but you do want to set yourself up for success where possible. And this can be done by trying to address, reduce, plan around and accommodate as many barriers as possible.

As an example, one of my barriers to exercise is that 99 per cent of the times I lie on my exercise mat, my annoying yet adorable little Chihuahua will try to sit on me and play with my hair tie or exercise bands/balls. Ways to address this are as follows:

- Enjoy the chaotic company; it makes things fun, and when he isn't there, I do miss him.
- If I want a more peaceful workout, I can time it to coincide with a distraction like his dinner/nap time.
- Explain to my fiancé (who exercises in a gym with no Chihuahuas) that I would also love to experience a peaceful workout, and perhaps he could help by occupying said dog (who is also half his).

As you can see from this silly but nevertheless very real example, solutions can seemingly be quite obvious, but often – when you are perhaps overtired, stressed, busy, in pain, in a bad mood and so on – you do not think logically in the moment. However, taking the time to pre-empt a situation gives you some tools in your belt to manage it when it arises.

The table opposite outlines some common barriers to exercise and how you might approach them.

Barrier	Why this may stop you	Questions to ask yourself when this happens
Pain*	Your pain levels are high which makes you unsure whether to exercise	• Notice and listen to your pain. What do you think your body is telling you? • Does exercise make this type of pain worse? • Can you try an exercise that normally feels good for your body and you feel comfortable doing? • Is there a way you can help to manage your pain before exercising – for example, pain relief, heat packs, pain-management strategies? • Is there a time in the day you find your pain levels are lower or when you feel your best?
Fatigue**	Feeling so exhausted you cannot contemplate starting to exercise or move your body in any way	• Can you set a timer for five minutes and try some movement? If after five minutes you feel worse (or no better), then stop and rest. If you feel ok, you may choose to carry on. • If five minutes feels too much, can you pick one exercise you can do right where you are, for just a minute or two? If this feels ok, you might be able to pick another one. • Can you assess what type of fatigue you are feeling? What do you think your body needs in this moment and could movement help? • Do you need a rest day today?

Barrier	Why this may stop you	Questions to ask yourself when this happens
Nausea	Movement can make nausea feel worse	• Can you time movement with when you have taken medication? • Would changing when you eat or drink around exercise help reduce the nausea? • If you chose one position, such as sitting upright or supported sitting, would this make movement more possible with nausea? • Can you reduce the intensity of your activity, so it feels more manageable with nausea?
Having to get changed	The energy required, or even the thought of needing to get changed, stops you exercising	• Can you exercise in what you are wearing? • Or can you adapt your exercise plan to what you are wearing? • Next time, can you either lay out clothes earlier or wear them to begin with? • Can you break up getting changed with another task, and then come back to exercise later, so it feels less overwhelming overall?
Having to go somewhere to exercise	The energy or thought of needing to move from where you are stops you exercising	• Can you change your plan to exercise where you are, whether in bed on the sofa – wherever? • Can you do the activity at home, rather than having to leave the house? • Can you break down the journey to the gym by pairing it with another errand or something fun like getting a hot drink afterwards?

Barrier	Reframe	Suggestions
Being too busy with work	Not having enough time in the day to exercise	• Can you exercise before or after work – even if only for ten to fifteen minutes? • Would lunchtime allow you some time for movement? • Can you fit in 'movement snacks' throughout the day – for example, micro-movement breaks of a few minutes at a time? • Can you work longer one day and less the next to free up time for exercise? • What can you do on your day off?
Having to care for a child (or pet)	You haven't got much time to yourself to exercise	• Can you include them in your exercises and make it fun for them, too? • Can you set them up in the same room as you with an activity and manage a short period of time then? • Can you look at the structure of your day and see if you can make space to give yourself time to exercise?
Needing to prioritise household tasks	You haven't got enough energy for both, so you do the housework	• Firstly, this still counts as physical activity, so no guilt needed! • Can you be mindful with **how** you move as you go about your tasks? • Can you add in some standing exercises while in the kitchen, like heel raises or leg lifts? • Can you add mobility movements on to the end of your tasks to help wind down your body at the end? • Can you delegate any of your tasks or re-assign as a priority to give yourself more space for your own movement?

*A note on pain

Pain is a big one. So big that it has its own chapter (Chapter 12) – because understanding the role pain plays, both physically and mentally, is important. Ridiculous phrases, such as 'no pain, no gain' and the mentality of pushing through the pain are not only wrong but can be harmful, too. Instead, we want to work with our bodies to help them feel safe through movement and, in turn, we can gradually increase our capacity for what we can do. We will go into more detail as to how this can be done, but firstly, it's about understanding that pain does not mean an automatic 'no' to exercise (although in some cases it may be). Asking yourself the following questions allows you to have a better understanding of your pain and how you could work with it to move your body, and maybe even help it:

- Is this a new sensation or something I have experienced before?
- If this is something I have experienced before, did it get worse when I moved?
- If I begin to move from the sofa/bed and start getting ready to exercise, does it feel worse?
- What can I use from my pain-management toolbox (see p. 225) to help manage this pain?
- Can I modify what I had planned to do to make it feel more manageable?

My new favourite motto is from movement therapist Jeannie Di Bon and it goes 'no pain, no strain'. The aim is to work with your body, rather than push it past what it can cope with.

**A note on fatigue

Another huge factor which has its own chapter (Chapter 11). The main tool here is pacing and how you set up your exercise regime to prevent a boom-and-bust approach. One thing that can be hard to identify (especially if you are resting in bed or on the sofa) is: are you really so fatigued that your body does need to rest or are you feeling lethargic and in a slump because you haven't moved your body in a while? It can be helpful to try and tune into your fatigue and think what your body needs. If you are unsure, the strategies in the table above can help you to see if you can do some movement, rather than none. Sometimes, when fatigued, starting can feel like the hardest part – just getting on your mat or on your bike or out the door. But starting and seeing how you feel can enable you to judge whether you just needed some help to get going or, you really are exhausted, and rest is what you need.

Caution: if your body is giving you all the signs it is fatigued, then it is important to listen. Ignoring and pushing past this will just perpetuate the boom-and-bust cycle and can cause more harm. Exercise can be harmful for anyone with severe chronic fatigue syndrome, myalgic encephalomyelitis or post-viral fatigue syndromes like long Covid (covered in Chapter 5).

Living with an autoimmune condition means symptoms act as extra barricades, so that even starting to exercise feels like an obstacle course. But the better we understand each potential barricade, the more we can work with it to get to where we want to be. The most important part is being self-compassionate throughout the process. Just as we are trying to be kind to our bodies and work with our symptoms, we need to be kind to our minds, too – we are trying our best.

Contraindications to exercise

Sometimes we can be too brave for our own good, as we are used to putting up with so many symptoms and high pain levels. So it is important to know how to assess when exercise will not be helpful for the body, and when rest and/or medical assessment are needed before easing back into it.

Should I always check with my doctor before starting to exercise?

You should have clearance from a health professional before starting a new form of exercise if you have a health condition (gyms, fitness professionals or online exercise programmes usually advise this). However, since access to a medical team can be a challenge and time with your doctors is limited, this may not always be possible. Plus, 'Is it safe for me to exercise?' is a question that is unlikely to be answered fully by your doctor – because it depends on the intensity, level and type of exercise you may be starting with and they are unlikely to have the time or knowledge to go through all these variables and apply them to your personal situation in the course of an appointment, which has probably already covered a myriad other issues.

I feel that there are already enough natural obstacles to exercise with chronic illness, and adding in a further step in the form of medical clearance can raise that barrier so high that it puts people off altogether. In a way, the general instruction to speak to your doctor before starting a new exercise regime is a medicalisation of movement and perhaps makes you feel you have even less control in making decisions about your own body. My mission is to encourage you to become an expert on movement and use exercise to enhance your life. As part of that learning, you may want to draw on your doctor's experience and expertise, but, ultimately, the goal is for you to be in tune with whatever movement fits with how you feel. Having said that, it is also imperative that you are safe, so be sure to follow any advice or precautions set by your medical team.

To set yourself up for success when starting to add in exercise, whether on your own or with any trainer you may work with, the questions below will help to ensure that you begin with the right type of exercise and level for you.

The PAR-Q (physical activity readiness questionnaire) is a useful screening tool that fitness professionals use to assess people's safety for exercise (see Resources p. 236). The questionnaire, comprising seven questions relating to general health, is designed to highlight where additional medical clearance or advice are needed (for example, with heart conditions or medication complications) from a doctor or qualified exercise professional, so reducing the barriers many face to adding in more physical activity. If you answer no to all seven questions, you are cleared for physical activity; if you answer yes to any of them, it does not necessarily mean that you cannot exercise, but it is recommended that you work with a professional to fill out a more detailed form (the PAR-Q+) with further questions to determine more about your health condition/s.

When might be a time *not* to exercise?

1. When a doctor says no

It is quite rare for a medical team to say an absolute no to exercise, so if they do, you should listen to their advice. In the past, bedrest was a valid treatment and exercise was more frequently forbidden. However, nowadays, research shows movement is essential for our health. Even after invasive surgery, most hospitals will have you up and walking as soon as you are medically stable and your pain is controlled. Rather than advising against exercise completely, it is more likely that your medical team will recommend certain restrictions, such as not letting your heart rate or blood pressure go over a particular number, or to only weight bear for a specified time and so on. In the event that they do say no, it is important to understand why, as well as how to get clearance (and when) and any ongoing limitations.

2. New, unexplained symptoms

Particularly heart conditions, such as increased heart rate, new arrhythmias or new respiratory symptoms, like increased shortness of breath, new pain that you are unable to manage with your usual tools or new episodes of dizziness, balance issues and so on. Anything that feels very different from what you normally cope with should be explored before you continue to exercise. This is when I say trust your gut: if something doesn't feel right, get it checked out. We usually know our bodies very well, even if we cannot always explain what is happening, so if something feels off and it seems like it might impact your ability to exercise, see if you can get some advice first.

3. Unstable health and conditions

This will be relative to whatever your current symptoms and diagnosis already are. The nature of autoimmune conditions is that symptoms fluctuate and the stability of your health can change. However, a significant deterioration in your function and/or an increase in symptoms would suggest you need to check in with your team, who should be there to offer you support and advice at such times. Feeling less well than 'usual' does not always mean you have to stop everything; often, you just need to reconsider your activity balance. With things like an unstable heart condition or unstable diabetes, for example, it is useful to have a plan in place to help you know when or how to exercise safely (we will cover how to adapt exercise to ever-changing conditions in Chapter 10). Equally, this can be used with conditions where you experience flares, so you have a plan in place for who to contact and what to do when this happens.

4. Acute illness

With many of us having compromised immune systems, we often get sick with common colds and viruses, too. Getting any kind of cold/bug/virus alongside everything you are already coping with can feel frustrating and unfair, but it is so important to recognise the impact on your body and not try to push through. The idea of 'sweating it out' is outdated and it is now thought best to rest during the acute stage of illness, especially if you think it could be Covid or a flu, have a fever or symptoms below the neck, such as extra fatigue, aches, coughing or upset stomach. If you have symptoms above the neck, such as congestion, headache, earache, research shows that exercise does not cause harm. However, I'd only recommend low-level exercise and mobility movements that can help with symptoms and boost circulation. Of course, low level to one person can mean high level to the next, so when in doubt, stick to breathwork and a few repetitions of gentle movements that may help to combat any pain or tightness from being curled up resting.

If you have just had symptoms of a cold, then usually, after two to three days, you can ease back into things as you feel able. Some movement, like gentle walks, can help to ease the tail end of congestion. If you had a fever, it is recommended to wait longer – five to seven days after it has lifted – before you return to exercise. Advice is similar if you have had the flu, a virus or anything that wiped you out for longer than a normal cold – wait until your symptoms are better and then give yourself an extra day or two before you return to exercise. Depending on how long you were sick for and your recovery, you will probably need to adjust the intensity and duration by only doing 30 to 50 per cent of what you managed pre-illness.

5. Acute Covid

I don't think many of us have managed to avoid it, but if you have, congratulations! As with other colds, research has found that exercising regularly prior to catching Covid is associated with a lower likelihood of adverse outcomes, as well as less severe symptoms and shorter recovery times. It is also an important tool in your recovery. However, as with other viruses, rest is recommended while experiencing acute symptoms. For anyone who has had mild Covid, current guidelines suggest ten days of deliberate rest (i.e. not exercising and reducing functional tasks where possible) and at least seven symptom-free days before gradually returning to exercise. With moderate to severe Covid (including if you were hospitalised), it is recommended that you see your medical team once symptoms have eased for an assessment before returning to exercise. Red flags for not exercising post-Covid include chest pain, out-of-proportion breathlessness and tachycardia (high heart rate), along with post-exertional symptom exacerbation (see next point). I have found from working with clients with autoimmune conditions that Covid often exacerbates their usual symptoms. Where this is the case, recovery may take longer or additional medical management may be required.

6. **Chronic fatigue syndrome (CFS)/myalgic encephalomyelitis (ME) and long Covid**

   Fatigue is a common symptom for those living with autoimmune conditions and is classified as chronic after experiencing it for six months. CFS/ME is a separate, complex, multisystem disease which is different from chronic fatigue as a symptom with specific diagnostic criteria. One of the diagnostic criteria for CFS, ME and post-viral syndromes like long Covid is the hallmark symptom of post-exertional malaise (PEM), which is the worsening of symptoms following physical or mental exertion and can vary in severity and duration but can last from days to months. They are often known as post-infectious fatigue syndromes, frequently starting after an infectious illness (now including long Covid), with symptoms lasting beyond the acute infectious stage. It is important to note that with all these conditions, there is a spectrum of severity, from mild (such as undertaking some daily activities but having to pace or carefully manage) to very severe, being bedridden and having to live in sensory deprivation (inability to tolerate any light or sound).

Exercise can be a vital tool in the management of CFS/ME and can help to prevent deconditioning, which can exacerbate symptoms (although deconditioning is not the cause of these conditions). However, exercise is not recommended for those with ME/CFS or long Covid when their condition is unstable. You need to be in a position of relative stability at a level of baseline function (more of which in the next chapter) and then work with an exercise specialist who can tailor your movement without triggering PEM. (Note: graded exercise therapy is no longer a recommended treatment and is not safe for those with CFS/ME.)

I hope all this has made it simpler to gauge when it is not safe to exercise. It is tricky to give definite answers, as so much is down to how you as an individual present, your medical management and changing recommendations due to the lack of research in exercising with autoimmunity. If in doubt, get help from a movement specialist and/or check in with your medical team. You need to feel safe to exercise, and the peace of mind you get from being given the green light really helps.

6

How to exercise with autoimmune conditions

This is the big one. The conundrum that is most likely the reason why you've chosen to read this particular book and the main reason I am writing it.

Exercise is good for you. This is a loud, and frequently imparted message. But while there are so many different voices telling us to exercise, far fewer give clear instructions or guidelines about how to go about it with an autoimmune condition. Protocols can be too simplistic or too complicated and assume energy levels, resilience and recovery far beyond your reality. So it is completely understandable if you are finding it hard to know how to actually do it.

There isn't one magic way to exercise that suits everybody, works instantly and cures autoimmune conditions. If this was the case, I could simply stand (or more likely sit) and point you in the right direction. Instead, it is more of an individual journey. I spend a lot of time answering questions on social media with 'It depends'. And that's because we all have to adapt to our specific needs and bodies, while factoring in what we enjoy, what fits in with our lifestyle and our 'whys' and goals.

Understanding activity

My approach to supporting clients to exercise is to keep things as simple as possible. We want to help you find a way to move more, but in a way that stays within your body's comfort zone. So the first task is to identify your current baseline. This is probably the hardest part, and the reason why so many people living with auto-immunity struggle to find a consistent way to exercise.

Here are some definitions to help you label different types of activity:

- **Physical activity** = any body movement that increases energy expenditure above resting levels – for example, all everyday activities, leisure and recreation, sport, exercise
- **Exercise** = a form of physical activity, often differentiated by being something 'structured or planned', like a game of tennis, a gym workout, Pilates, etc.; I often call it formal movement or formal exercise
- **Functional activity** = activities of daily living, such as getting out of bed in the morning, standing, getting dressed, cooking a meal, cleaning; most healthy people do not realise functional activity uses energy, and it certainly does not drain their reserves, but for those of us living with energy-limiting conditions, functional activity can be really challenging and leave little space for formal exercise

Your activity cup

I find visualising an activity cup a useful tool when adding more movement to our lives. Imagine that you start every day with a cup. Whenever you do some form of physical activity, whether formal or functional, you add water to your cup. If your cup becomes too full, it will overflow. And an overflow will likely trigger symptoms over the following few days.

Everyone's cup is a different size. A healthy, robust person has a huge cup. For them, the energy required for showering and drying off would be represented by a tiny drop in their enormous cup. It would make little difference to their activity plans for the rest of their day. A person living with fatigue, however, will have a much smaller cup. And simply taking a shower could fill up their cup for the day.

It would be easier if your cup was the same size every day, but for those living with chronic illness it varies day to day. Successive busy days can mean the cup gets smaller and smaller, as the fatigue builds. Other factors like stress, sleep, nutrition, medication and the overall stability of your condition can also affect your cup's capacity. Consequently, on some days a particular activity will feel ok, but on others, the same thing will cause your cup to overflow and wipe you out.

Chronic-illness activity cups fill quickly and drain slowly. It can take two to three days post activity for your cup to empty again. So you need to think about what is going into it over several days because rest isn't going to be an instant fix, which means pacing across the week is necessary. Still, frustratingly, no matter how carefully you plan your days, life throws up unexpected events: your train is cancelled, the clinic runs late and suddenly you have been out of the house for five hours instead of one. Your cup then overflows, recovery is a struggle and emotionally, you feel battered.

It can be frustrating and limiting having a tiny cup, constantly needing to choose between functional activities or formal exercise. On high-symptom days, even the basic functional activities alone are too much, meaning that fun or anything else that's helpful for your health are totally off your menu.

Understanding your activity cup can help you to add movement into your routine at the right intensity, level and time for you. It might be that you can start with a few arm or leg movements in bed, as that's all you can manage. The key is to prioritise movement before your cup's capacity has been taken up by your usual everyday functional activity. Consistently prioritising a safe amount of movement by not constantly overfilling your cup in the short term can give you a bigger cup in the long term. Conversely, not prioritising your needs and constantly overfilling your cup, boom-and-bust style, will lead to a smaller cup and being able to cope with less and less over time.

Achieving this balance requires mindfulness. It requires you to look at every part of your day and see which things can be delegated, are non-essential or can be done less frequently. You are going to prioritise your own needs. You are trying to create space in your activity cup, and within that space, you are you going to move, you are going to become stronger and fitter, so that in the future you can do more of what you want to do.

A useful exercise here is to write down everything that's filling up your cup – for example, gardening, cognitive tasks, caring for a pet or child, medical care, laundry, self-care, hygiene, shopping, hobbies, socialising . . .

This helps you to see just how much you are doing. A lot of my clients tell me that exercise just does not work or that it always makes them feel worse. Exercise gets the blame for all the symptoms they experience. However, the real problem is that everything else they are trying to do is filling their activity cup. Yes, exercise may be the activity that causes their cup to overflow, but that does not mean it has been bad for them. If you feel your cup is already full from just managing your daily activities, you can probably understand why adding in exercise and expecting your already fatigued body to cope with it is not going to work.

Sometimes you don't have a choice with your commitments, whether for your family or work and that is tough – but that's just life. If this is the case for you, take hope from the fact that making even small choices that create a little bit of extra space in your activity cup can allow the addition of some movement. This might mean adapting functional tasks (such as using a stool in the kitchen, asking for help with strenuous tasks like carrying washing loads or vacuuming). Or you can also look to gain space for movement throughout the day by adding in more rest breaks (we will cover more about pacing in Chapter 10). Looking at the whole picture like this helps you to add exercise in a way that won't make your fatigue and symptoms worse.

Your baseline

Ideally, we would live each day, being as busy as we can manage, neither overdoing it nor hibernating, and being able to sustain that activity level, whatever it is, day after day.

Take some time to consider a day that is well paced for you. It's probably a day that goes to plan with no unexpected events and you can manage your normal routine. Focus on your average day here.

Ask yourself: would a day like this be something you can repeat every day? If you can answer yes, then this shows it is sustainable for you – this is your baseline measurement, where your activity cup is full of meaningful things for you, but it is not overspilling. Your usual amount of rest and recovery means you start the day with your usual level of symptoms. If you answered no, it isn't repeatable or is only repeatable every other day, it is likely you are trying to overfill your cup.

For example, a baseline day for me means I can get out of bed at my usual time, manage my usual routine, work three to four hours, do a couple of chores, make meals and fit in some form of exercise for thirty minutes. This day still includes rest and self-care activities to help me manage, but the overall activity level is sustainable for me on average. If I have an infection, that means I have to lower my activity level to below baseline. I may be slower getting out bed, I will do the bare minimum in terms of functional tasks around the house, my partner may take over the dog walk and cooking and I may do less work or be unable to work at all. I know this is only short term, so it doesn't mean my baseline has changed at this stage – just that I am currently below my baseline. If, however, the infection lingers (which it often does) and my lupus starts to flare as a result, or maybe I end up in hospital and become more unwell, this starts to have a bigger impact on my health. As the weeks start to add up and I become deconditioned, my 'usual' routine is no longer achievable, and I would then say my baseline has dropped and it may look quite different. At the other end of the spectrum, if I have a smooth run for a few months and can be consistent with my exercise, nutrition and routines, I can improve my baseline such that my 'average' day might include a higher level of physical activity.

When you add in exercise, you want to do it in such a way that you can maintain your baseline. If after adding in exercise, you have worsening symptoms and struggle to do the remaining baseline activities you can normally manage, then you've probably undertaken too much activity.

It is not an exact science. Therefore, when you first introduce movement it is important to be conservative, to be sure you remain within your baseline level, taking small steps forward, rather than repeating previous patterns of going too hard and needing days to recover.

Noticing your baseline can be incredibly empowering, preventing any negative impact on how you feel and function. By understanding both your activity cup and your baseline, you can adapt and create space for movement, so building your strength and resilience.

Sit, stand and walk

You can also look at your baseline for specific activities. When answering the questions below, think about what you could comfortably manage on a typical day without it impacting your other activities or symptoms, as we discussed above – so how long you can safely sit, stand or walk without your symptoms flaring either on that day or subsequent days.

1. **What is your current tolerance for sitting upright?** I, for example, can sit in a chair for two hours without needing a break. For some of my clients, however, this may be minutes. It can also be helpful to break down this question further by separating how long you can sit unsupported (meaning without back support) and how long you can sit supported (on a chair with a back).

2. **What is your current tolerance for standing?** As an example, I often ask my clients if they had to stand completely still, how long could they manage? This will usually be measured in seconds or minutes – or maybe longer!

3. **What is your current tolerance for walking?** If you require mobility aids, such as a stick or a frame, it can be helpful

again to identify how long you can manage both with and without them. This can be measured in time or distance.

The answers to these questions will help you to assess your starting point for any exercise and also which type might be good to begin with. If your sitting tolerance is only a few minutes, lying sounds like a good position from which to start to move. If your walking tolerance is ten minutes, you're not going to start running just yet. If you are already doing some kind of activity or sport, it can be useful to also benchmark your tolerance for that – for example, 'I can cycle for ten minutes comfortably' or, 'I can play half a game of tennis – any more and I tend to flare the next day'. Trying to analyse and put it all into numbers can help take some of the guesswork out of how much is 'enough' and what is 'too much'.

When to add in exercise

Once you have a better idea of all the physical activity you are currently doing and your baseline and activity cup, you can look at when it might be possible to incorporate some movement into your lifestyle. Start with a look across your week and try to work out which days might be best to start. Ideally, you want to pick days that are not too close together at first, balancing your physical activity across a week. This is going to depend on where your current baseline is and what your functional activity looks like.

Example 1: Rachel lives with extreme fatigue and pain from lupus, while also managing chronic migraine, and has not been able to exercise for four years. She spends most of her time at home, either resting in bed or doing activities from the sofa. On Mondays she tries to meal prep for the week, and she has some help with house-work but cleans her bedroom herself. This is how we paced out her week to balance her goals for exercise, along with rest days and functional activities:

- Monday – mobility + meal prep
- Tuesday – strength
- Wednesday – rest
- Thursday – mobility + clean bedroom
- Friday – strength
- Saturday – rest
- Sunday – short walk

Example 2: Steven lives with ankylosing spondylitis (a type of arthritis) and struggles with stiffness and pain. He works full time and enjoys being active, but his baseline for tolerating formal exercise is currently low. He finds he is exhausted by Thursday/Friday, as his job is busy and stressful. He shares the load of household tasks and cooking with his partner. Here is Steven's ideal plan for his week to balance out commute, household tasks and exercise goals.

- Monday – walk to and from work, mobility exercises
- Tuesday – train to and from work, strength exercises
- Wednesday – walk to work, train home from work, yoga class at home
- Thursday – train to and from work, rest
- Friday – walk to and from work, rest (optional mobility)
- Saturday – longer walk or cycle with partner, some household chores
- Sunday – strength, household chores

The examples above illustrate a balance between functional activities (like housework), social and work commitments and formal exercise. This balance, with the inclusion of movement exercise, will help you to control your pain and symptoms without exacerbating them and work towards achieving goals.

Choosing between types of exercise

As soon as you refer to an autoimmune condition, yoga is usually mentioned – probably followed shortly after by turmeric or drinking celery juice. But the last thing anybody needs when living with a chronic condition is a 'wellness' expert suggesting baseless remedies. Do I sound frustrated? Well, I am – because it is daunting enough trying to pick between different types of exercise without having to unpick misleading and unfounded claims.

Within each genre – whether yoga, Pilates, fitness classes, gym regimes and more – there are many levels and the descriptions can be confusing and inconsistent. For instance, 'beginner' classes often last an hour and include lots of standing and planks. 'Low-impact' regimes can have you doing burpees and squats. As for the language I referred to earlier of 'push through', 'no gain without pain', 'you can do it' – this is alienating for all but the fittest among us. No wonder it is so difficult to choose between different types of exercise!

In truth, there is no one type of exercise you cannot do at all when living with an autoimmune illness – unless you have been explicitly told so by your doctor. Sometimes you cannot do things *right now*, but you can build up to them, which is really the same for anyone. An average person cannot just decide to do a marathon and run it straight away – they need months to prepare, train and build up to it. Equally, if you decide you want to try tennis, you cannot just play a full match without any training – or perhaps you can, but you may be more likely to injure yourself or flare afterwards. Our bodies need to prepare and become skilled at whatever task we want them to do. This reduces the risk of injury and prevents overdoing it.

Some types of exercise are easier to tailor to your condition than others. The easier types are those in which you can be in control of the variables, such as duration and intensity. Playing football, for example, requires lots of skills straight away, such as speed, agility, stability and stamina. Even for just a short time, the demands are high and lots of work off the pitch would be required to build up to playing the game. However, with something like hiking, you can gradually increase your stamina, the challenge of the terrain and the distance over time.

Of course, you need to enjoy the activity you are choosing. So no matter how suitable hiking is as an activity to build stamina and strength, it's no use to you if you hate doing it – and, by extension, it will not be good for you either. You will start to resent it and form negative associations with exercise because of it. I don't believe you have to love every second, but fundamentally enjoying the type of exercise you have chosen has been shown to help with long-term effectiveness. I also feel that when trying to rewrite your beliefs around movement, away from pain or negative past experiences, picking something you enjoy can help to reframe it in a more positive way.

The type of movement you choose also depends on where you can exercise and what is accessible to you. A lot of my clients start with exercising at home, as this means the impact on their energy is minimal. It doesn't require travelling anywhere and you don't have to worry about what you look like/what you are wearing – I regularly end up exercising in my pyjamas or non-activewear, as for me, getting changed can use up energy that I'd rather save for the exercise itself. Exercising at home doesn't call for a lot of equipment, so it can also be low cost. At a minimum, all you need is a small space and maybe a mat or something comfortable for the floor. You can then add some light weights and/or exercise bands if you want to make things more enjoyable or challenging. Exercise bikes are also a great, relatively affordable tool, and you can get folding ones that take up less space. There are also several brands that make portable or foldable treadmills that can be really useful, especially if the temperature outside is a barrier to walking.

The time you spend exercising can be quite short when you start out or when you are building back up – for example, a five-minute cycle or a fifteen-minute strength programme. This can make gyms uneconomical as they usually don't give discounts for people with disabilities or those who cannot make as much use of the facilities as others. It can also be a lot of effort to travel somewhere to exercise for such a short time, and stacking the journey with exercising can use up your precious energy resources, leaving less for the main event. Exercising at home also means you can be even more flexible with timing, grabbing a few moments rather than having to plan it as a big part of the day. However, some people do prefer to have a set place to go, like a gym, whether in their building, if they are lucky enough to have one on site, or somewhere close by. Sometimes the act of going somewhere else helps to initiate exercise, rather than procrastinating at home. Wherever you choose to practise movement, it is also worth bearing in mind the additional energy that may be required – for example, swimming also involves getting changed and showering, which increases the demands of that activity.

Now that we have considered how best to approach exercise and add it into your sustainable routine, in the next chapter, we will move on to the different types available to you.

7

Types of exercise

These days, we are spoiled for options of how to move our bodies – and this can be exciting or daunting, depending on how you look at it. So in this chapter we will look at what each type is and how it could be helpful for you.

Strength training

Strength is defined as the ability to exert force on an external resistance. This can be done with weights, weight machines, resistance bands or just with your own body weight. People tend to think that lifting weights is about putting on muscle bulk or 'toning up', however, the WHO recommends 'muscle-strengthening activities involving major muscle groups on two or more days a week' for health benefits. Studies show that just thirty to sixty minutes of strength training a week (if targeting all the major muscle groups) was found to be the optimal dose of strength with the most benefits for our health.

Strength training has been shown to be effective for reducing lower-back pain and helping with pain related to arthritis and fibromyalgia. The best combination when it comes to preventing or managing chronic health conditions seems to be a mix of strength and aerobic training, but for those reintroducing exercise, strength is the best place to start, as it also helps with activities of daily living (such as picking shopping bags up off the floor).

The great thing with strength training is that you can start really small, with supported body-weight movements like the ones in this book. Once you've mastered this, you can begin to demand more of the muscles by changing the positions you use, working with gravity to help you or against it to make a movement more challenging. You can increase the load on your muscles by adding in more resistance, using bands, weights and so on. And you can start by keeping the repetitions (the number of times you repeat a movement) low and building up the sets (a group of repetitions), as well as playing around with rest and recovery times.

Exercise classes

There is a huge range of classes available now, both online and in person. A lot of my clients ask me, 'Can I get back to yoga?' or, 'Can I go back to my boxing class?' or similar, and my typical answer is, 'It depends'. Not wanting to sound like a broken record, it depends on what will fit in your activity cup or within your baseline (see pp. 56–61). Is this something you have worked back up towards doing or will you be diving straight in and trying a sixty-minute high-intensity class? How helpful is the instructor in providing adaptations and tailoring to the individual? How much can you modify it to work with your body, rather than pushing it beyond its limitations, just to keep up with the class? Are there different levels you can take? Could you perhaps do half a class and build up the amount of time you do?

Group training can be great, giving clients a chance to keep exercise varied, while staying accountable with others. A study found group classes led to a significant decrease in stress and increase in physical, mental and emotional quality-of-life scores compared to exercising alone or not at all. However, if you are someone with a chronic condition and unable to keep up with others in class, perhaps being the only one who needs to adapt exercises or ask for modifications can leave you feeling a mixture of emotions, potentially comparing yourself to those around you or feeling frustrated because of what your body is unable to do. This is especially so if you are grappling with the acceptance of your current physical abilities and trying not to compare them with how they were in the past.

There are some great classes, including healthcare-run (like falls-prevention) or condition-specific ones, which bring you all the benefits of exercising in a group, alongside others who really 'get it' – they are literally designed for you! A study on classes for patients with ankylosing spondylitis showed that group exercise was more effective in a hospital clinic than home-based exercises. Sadly, however, these types of health-specific classes are often hard to access or have limited capacity and are often for a set period – a six-week course, for example.

There are also circuit formats or classes that are high intensity or a mixture of strength and cardiovascular exercise. These can be great to mix things up or for trying different types of exercise. However, it can also be hard to stay within your baseline, especially with a fun, fast-paced class, where you might be experiencing an endorphin high or encouraged by an instructor to 'push harder' than you planned to. These classes may be a form of exercise you can work up to, but if you struggle with heart-rate regulation, fatigue or pain, I would not recommend starting with them.

Pilates

Pilates is my personal favourite. It can be done on a one-to-one basis or in a class format, with or without equipment. Pilates is a full-body form of exercise that, through controlled movements, builds strength, flexibility, stability and body awareness. It was created by Joseph Pilates, who suffered with health conditions as a child. He devised a conditioning group of exercises to help support his own health and then, during World War I, he helped injured soldiers to recover through exercises he then called 'contrology'. He later opened a studio and helped dancers and others who needed rehabilitation. He focused on key principles, which are still used as the foundations of Pilates today: concentration, breathing, control, centring and precision.

Mat Pilates is just you on a mat, maybe using equipment like a small ball, bands or magic circle (circular resistance ring). Reformer Pilates is done on a sliding carriage that's suspended on a frame, with springs. A lot of the movements are similar to those on the mat, but due to the springs, you have different levels of resistance. Many people believe reformer Pilates is automatically more challenging than the mat version, but sometimes the mat can be harder, as there is nothing to assist you. With both, you can start at a very low level and then ramp it all the way up, where even the strongest person's legs will be shaking. This is why I love it as a form of movement, as it can still be fun and challenging, but in a supportive, low-impact way for your body. I also teach bed Pilates on Actively Autoimmune Studio, which can, as the name suggests, be done from your bed. I have had people join the live class while in hospital, which shows just how gentle a baseline you can start from.

Yoga

Yoga is a great option for moving with an autoimmune condition, as there are multiple types and ways to modify your practice to work with your body. Many people say they cannot do yoga or are 'bad' at it because they are not flexible. But flexibility is not required, nor is it the only benefit. Depending on the type of yoga, regular practice can improve strength, range of motion, co-ordination and cardiovascular function. It can also help to reduce stress, help with anxiety, depression, chronic pain and improve sleep quality. Yoga is used as a complementary therapy for many conditions; it has been shown to decrease inflammation in rheumatoid arthritis and reduce fatigue for those with multiple sclerosis.

Vinyasa yoga is probably the best known, and is a series of flows of different postures, using your breath. Depending on the teacher or type of vinyasa, it can be quite intense, but it can also be modified using equipment, such as blocks, or done in a chair, for seated yoga. Hatha yoga is similar to vinyasa but tends to be slower, holding postures for longer and building up your foundations of strength and breathwork. Yin yoga is slower again, where you tend to hold postures for typically between three and five minutes (I would not recommend this for beginners, as it uses a passive range of movement for which a certain level of skill is required to avoid irritating inflamed joints). Restorative yoga is my favourite; like yin, it involves holding postures with minimal movement, but it uses blankets and bolsters to support the body and help you to relax and rest.

With yoga, it really depends on your teacher and how they can help you to modify it as needed. As with all exercise, it may take time to find the style that works with your body.

Tai chi and qi gong

These are mind–body movement practices that help with health and wellness and have roots in ancient Chinese tradition. Both have been found to aid with the balance of the autonomic nervous system, helping to bring the body into its parasympathetic state (rest and digest – see p. 224), which has proven effective for those living with a chronic-pain condition. Along with the usual benefits of regular movement, some research suggests that tai chi and qi gong have a positive impact on the immune system's function and inflammatory processes, although further studies are needed.

Tai chi is often described as 'meditation in motion'. Focusing on slow, controlled movements combined with deep breathing in anything from short sessions to more advanced, longer ones, it aims to improve the *qi* (also called *chi*, which is the energy force in our bodies). Qi gong overlaps with tai chi but focuses on a series of just eight movements; it is slower and often easier, due to repetitions of the same movements over and over. Both are low-impact forms of movement, so they are gentle on the joints, and there is a big focus on balance, again, making them ideal for those with chronic conditions. It is often done in standing and holding static poses which may be a challenge for those with orthostatic intolerance.

Boxing

Boxing is a great form of aerobic activity, whether practised alone, one-to-one with a trainer or in a group setting. You do not have to hit anyone or risk getting punched yourself, as you will either do air punches or use punching bags/targets. It is a fun form of exercise, especially if traditional cardio/aerobic activities do not appeal. However, if you suffer with pain or swelling in your upper limbs, then using a punching bag may not be a good starting point for you. It is possible to modify by focusing on air punches, sitting down and including more rest breaks, but its's also easy to 'overdo it', pushing you into your anaerobic zone (see p. 205), which may increase fatigue and inflammation, as well as raising cortisol levels, which can contribute to a flare.

Aerobic activity

Aerobic activity, often known as cardio or cardiovascular fitness, is defined by the American College of Sports Medicine (ACSM) as any activity using large muscle groups, that can be maintained continuously and is rhythmic in nature. Activating muscles in this way aims to improve the ability of the heart, lungs and muscles to utilise oxygen. This generally includes activities such as walking, running, cycling, swimming and HIIT (high-intensity interval training).

I find people are often all or nothing with aerobic exercise. They either think that's the only form of exercise they need to do or are terrified of it. So it's especially helpful to address any prior beliefs, thoughts or expectations you may have on how this 'should' look or feel. Many of the clients I work with push way too hard with their cardiovascular exercise, go into that dreaded boom-or-bust pattern and then declare they can no longer exercise because it makes their autoimmune condition worse. And it is not their fault – after all, exercise is still advertised with huge a bias towards fit, healthy and young people, rarely shining a light on the often less exciting, slower-paced cardio that most of the population would gain optimum benefit from. But it may well be that that your cardio involves little to no sweating and Lycra is most definitely not required.

As mentioned earlier, the WHO recommends two and a half to five hours of moderate aerobic activity a week (which can include activities like a brisk walk, golf, mowing the lawn) or one and a quarter to two and a half hours of vigorous activity, such as jogging, cycling or football. Or a combination of the two. This translates to thirty minutes of aerobic activity for five days a week. This may sound overwhelming if you are just starting out, but don't panic. The aim is to slowly build up to do what you can manage, keeping to your baseline. Most of my clients with autoimmune conditions probably stay in the moderate-intensity category, but that isn't to say you can't work towards including more vigorous types of activity. Understanding how hard your body is working and controlling that can be a helpful way of both pacing yourself and staying within your body's baseline or what it can tolerate. You can then start to play around with adding in more through changing variables and working your body harder in a slow and gradual way.

Types of aerobic activity

Aerobic activity includes anything that gets your heart pumping oxygenated blood more quickly around your body. It aims to improve your cardiorespiratory fitness in that it helps your heart and lungs to be more efficient.

Static cycling

Static indoor cycling is one of my favourite ways to build up stamina, both for myself and my clients. This is because on the bike you can control your speed, resistance, the temperature of the room you are in, how upright you are and your upper-body position. The downside, of course, is that you need access to an indoor bike!

If you have a condition such as dysautonomia or symptoms of dizziness, it's recommended to start with a reclining bike. Many people with joint pain, especially knee or hip pain, also find this more comfortable at first. I would put my upright bike against a wall and pop a cushion behind my back and the wall, to provide some lumbar support (this helped me when I was weaker). You can also buy static pedals which you can use with any chair. They can be annoying to position correctly (I recommend having them against a wall, so that when you pedal, they stay put and cannot move further away from you), but are a more affordable and compact option. I have clients who use them at their desk or who sit watching TV in the evenings, pedalling away.

Even if you know you've been able to cycle 10k in the past or think that a few minutes is too easy, we want to gradually build up here, working with your body.

Warm-up and cool-down on the bike

Arguably the most important part of any exercise, but even more so for people with chronic illness, is to gradually prepare the body for the part where you work harder and then slowly wind down the body in readiness to stop. So much of chronic illness is about dysregulation, whether that be the immune system, nervous system and pain – we are trying to support the body to relearn how to work in this balanced way.

With the warm-up, you want to start with little to no resistance and begin by pedalling really slowly. With each minute you can increase the intensity, whether by pedalling slightly faster or increasing the resistance from one to two on the bike. The idea in this phase is to build up, so that you are at the desired intensity for your main section of the workout. With the cool-down, you do the opposite: every minute you drop the intensity, slowing down or reducing the resistance, so you gradually bring yourself to a point of rest. This is important whether you are doing a five-minute or thirty-minute cycle.

For the main section of your cycle, it depends on what your goal is. If you want to focus on building your stamina and managing longer cycles, you may focus on maintaining a steady pace throughout. Or maybe you want to stay with shorter cycles, and instead play with intensities, ramping it up and then recovering, otherwise known as interval training.

HOW TO ADD IN CYCLING

To start cycling, you want to start with an amount that you know you can manage – this could be based on the last time you cycled (for example, you comfortably managed ten minutes) or, if you are new to cycling or it has been a very long time since you were last on a bike, start with a very short duration (for example, five minutes). Each cycle, however short, must include a warm-up and cool-down section – so a five-minute cycle would break down into a two-minute warm-up, one-minute main cycle and two-minute cool-down. As you go along, check in with how you feel, as well as noting how you feel afterwards and over the following couple of days. If everything feels ok,

---

you can increase your time by one to two minutes each cycle. If, however, you felt it was hard work at any point during the cycle, you did not complete it or you felt worse afterwards, go back a step and repeat a previous level, until it feels easier. If you haven't got on your bike or cycled at all for more than five days, I recommend going back to your baseline cycle – one that you know you can comfortably complete.

As you progress, you can slowly increase your warm-up and cool-down (so they start to be between five and ten minutes long) and increase the middle section of your cycle (what we often call your base pace). To make it harder, you can start to work at different intensities, either using your target heart rate or your rating on the Borg RPE Scale (see p. 89). Generally, your base pace is around 2–3 out of 10 on the RPE scale and medium pace is 4–5 out of 10.

Outdoor cycling

Cycling outdoors may be a hobby or method of transport to get around. If possible, I recommend starting on an indoor bike to assess your baseline. If your baseline on an indoor bike is around 10 minutes, I would translate this to an actual bike as 5 minutes. This is because we have more to contend with when cycling outside including an increase in the cognitive load, with planning the journey, traffic, more neural stimulation from sound, sight, smells etc. It is also more physically demanding, as you have to factor in balance, different inclines, different road surfaces and so on. With an indoor bike, you have constant access to information to help guide how hard you are working, how long you have pedalled for and the distances/speed, making it easy to stay within what you know is your safe baseline. On an outdoor bike, you may not have any of this information, or it may be less easy to access during the cycle itself, which can lead to overdoing it. Plus, for many people, the enjoyment factor, especially of cycling outdoors or just pushing to get to where they want to be, means people go much further than they would normally do and then regret it afterwards. I have worked with many clients who transitioned from indoor to outdoor bike successfully by starting small and building up slowly. If you are patient in the early stages, you can get back to cycling as an activity if this is what you enjoy.

Walking

For those who can do it, walking is great way to work towards reaching the WHO's prescribed thirty minutes of moderate-to-vigorous physical activity on five or more days. It is relatively easy, accessible and comparatively low impact on your joints with low risk of injury. Walking is associated with all the usual health benefits of aerobic exercise, including reducing your risk of cardiovascular disease and preventing early death. Research shows it can improve sleep quality and help with weight management. It has also been shown to help reduce fatigue, pain and improve function in those with inflammatory conditions. Yet according to research on those living with fibromyalgia, pain and fatigue make it challenging to consistently go for walks. These symptoms are shared with other autoimmune conditions and are one of many reasons why those who have them are less physically active than the general population.

Before incorporating any 'formal' walks into your day, it's really important to assess *all* the walking that's currently in your activity cup. Step counts are a popular way to track your baseline, but if you do not have a device that does this (or if you feel it is something you may become unhealthily obsessed with) other markers, such as distance or time spent walking, can be just as helpful. Use whatever measure you find the easiest way to keep track. If you are struggling with low energy and high pain, it may be that we need to reduce your overall walking before we can build it up again.

You have probably heard of 10,000 steps as a daily goal, which sounds very hard and may be off-putting, especially if you struggle to walk even short distances around your home. So it's worth knowing that this benchmark was purely arbitrary, dreamed up by a Japanese company marketing a pedometer back in the 1960s, on the basis that they thought the Japanese character for 10k resembled a person walking.

We still do not have a magic number for the best benefits-to-steps ratio, but research has found that 7–8000 steps is enough to improve your health and lower your mortality rate compared to 4000. But even 4000 can sound overwhelming, depending on your current baseline. So the main takeaway here is that being active and moving is beneficial to your health, and the more steps you take, even if that is increasing from 1000 to 2000, the more it is going to help you. However, pushing your step count higher won't help you if by pushing it you are increasing your fatigue and feeling worse as a result. The balance of activity is key here, so if you do decide you want to progress with how far or how long you can walk, you need to do it slowly and incrementally to allow your body to cope with the increased load.

Start by working out your baseline ability to walk (time walking, number of steps, distance, etc.). For example, I can walk for fifteen minutes comfortably without flaring symptoms and could manage this consistently day in, day out, if I had to (which I do, as I have a Chihuahua, and every day I am thankful his legs are small and that a fifteen-minute walk is plenty for him). I could also push sixty to ninety minutes if I chose to, or had to, but this is not something I could do consistently. If I did, I would be exhausted and need to recover the rest of the day, so reducing my overall activity level. So my baseline would be fifteen minutes and that's what I would use as a basis for my walking programme.

Ideally, you still want to think about a warm-up and cool-down. What this looks like depends on your body, fitness level and what you find helpful. Some of my clients pick a few mobility exercises (see p. 155–80) before they start to help warm up. Others try to ensure the first few moments of their walk are at a slower pace, before getting their pace up for the middle section, then gradually slowing their pace again for the last phase. If you have one mode of walking – meaning all you can manage is a slow pace – don't worry too much about a warm-up/cool-down section.

The pace at which we walk dictates the benefits of walking. However, the important thing is what is sustainable for you. Similar to the cycling plan, it can be helpful to use the RPE scale while walking to assess how much effort you are using. For some clients, especially those with high fatigue or symptoms of dysautonomia, I recommend tracking heart rate, too, but this is optional. It is important to bring attention to how your body copes with walking and check in with yourself, but on the whole, I would value the joy of walking and relaxation, rather than overmedicalising and overthinking health, heart rate and symptoms.

Start with a five-minute walk. It may be within that walk or the others, as you build up, that you need to pause and rest. A rest may take the form of standing still or bracing (leaning against a wall or bench) or sitting down, if needed. If this is the case, the time is paused until you commence your walk again. Once you can get through the whole walk without needing to stop and rest, you are ready to try the same thing with the next increase in walking time. If you feel symptomatic during or after, you may want to return to the previous time or add in a rest break (or more rest breaks), as needed. Within each walk you can also vary the pace, starting off slowly for the first few minutes, then a slightly faster pace in the middle before ending slower again. You can also add intervals with longer walks – for example, a twenty-minute walk could comprise a five-minute warm-up, one minute slow pace, then one minute faster pace, with a cool-down walk for the last five minutes. If you are struggling to build up to a longer walk in one go, you could aim for two smaller walks a day, until your stamina and capacity allow you to build up to one longer walk, if that is your goal. It is all about what works for you and your lifestyle, with plenty of ways to vary pace, distance and energy requirements.

Hiking

Hiking is basically walking but at moderate difficulty, often for longer distances on paths or trails. Sometimes trails can be on uneven ground or have inclines. When training for this, you want to continue to increase your walking time/distance to your goal amount for your planned hike. You also need to factor in any inclines to prepare your body for this, too. This can be done by finding smaller hills to practise on, or you can walk on a treadmill and change the gradient to get used to this. Depending on the surface you are walking on, you may want to include balance exercises (see pp. 152–3) plus general strength training to support your joints. Often, the challenge with longer hikes is pacing across a number of hours/day, so the aim would be to increase your overall baseline of what you can walk – say, up to two or three hours – and then work on extra resilience for pushing past this for a one-off longer hike.

Running

For quite a lot of people, their ultimate goal is to get back to running, as perhaps it was something they enjoyed before their diagnosis. I think for many running represents being healthy and active, and I know personally the sense of freedom it brings. The benefits of running for our mental health are well researched and for our cardiovascular health, too, as it is a higher-intensity exercise which has been shown to have improved effects on mortality and disease risk over lower-intensity exercise. However, it can come at a cost, as running is often associated with injuries, usually from overuse, running too far or too fast, too soon. Injuries like stress fractures, tendon injuries and tripping and falling or rolling an ankle are also common.

I do not recommend running as your first option back to exercise following a diagnosis or time away from exercising. The increased load through the joints is often not a good idea with the pain and inflammation that can accompany autoimmune conditions. It also has high energy demands, with your heart rate remaining high throughout and, as such, it is not fatigue friendly. However, if it is something you are passionate about, you can work up to it, especially if you have previously been a runner and have experience in training.

As with everything else, the aim is to build up gradually, alternating with walking and gentle jogging, before incrementally increasing time spent running, speed and/or distance. It is generally advised to increase the amount by 10 per cent or less each week, but depending on how frequently you run and how you tolerate it, it may be worth increasing even more slowly. It is also important to include a warm-up. This could include dynamic stretching (see pp. 155–77) and movements that mimic what your body does and copes with while running, along with walking and then a slow jog to start off with. Your cool-down is important too, and may involve slowing your pace until you are walking and some static stretches to aid recovery.

There are several 'couch-to-5k' programmes which can be helpful for gradually building up your ability to run slowly. However, they are designed with healthy adults in mind, so don't worry if you have to start slower and smaller than the standard week 1 or take longer to progress through the weekly plans.

I recommend doing some strength training alongside your running, to help support your lower extremities in particular, and include functional and dynamic training specific to the skill of running to help with balance and co-ordination.

Aquatic exercise

Swimming is a great low-impact option to help improve strength and cardiovascular fitness. The buoyancy of the water supports your body and reduces pressure on the spine and joints, which can be helpful when you have pain in these areas. Research has shown that aquatic exercise can reduce pain and increase physical function in patients with lower-back pain, and 90 per cent of those participating in a study looking into the efficacy of aquatic exercise for lower-back pain improved within six months, irrespective of their ability to swim. There is also evidence suggesting that water-based exercise can improve wellness, symptoms and fitness in those with fibromylagia and help with disease activity in inflammatory arthritis. And there is some suggestion that any type of water-based activity can be helpful for mental-health management and may improve sleep and reduce pain in those with chronic musculoskeletal pain. Aquatic exercise training improved functional capacity, balance and perception of fatigue in women with MS and produced better pain and quality-of-life scores than land-based training for those with ankylosing spondylitis.

The negatives of swimming include the overall energy demands. As mentioned before, you have to factor in travelling to a pool, getting changed, getting in and out of the water, then showering and travelling home. Many people living with health problems are also economically disadvantaged, so swimming may be a challenge both in terms of affording access and proximity of a pool to where they live. For those with bladder and bowel conditions swimming can also present practical challenges and some people with allergies or skin sensitivities may also struggle with certain pool chemicals (for them, it can be worth researching different types of pool, such as saltwater vs chlorine).

Even walking or doing exercises in the water can be beneficial. You can also use a float to practise kicking up and down the pool. In terms of stroke, it's about doing what you feel most comfortable with. Most people choose freestyle/front crawl or breaststroke. Backstroke is also a great option, although it can be tough on your shoulders, so you could always just do backstroke kick.

For those in pain who find regular training a challenge, it can feel great to be in the water. Suddenly, your body seems lighter and it feels so much easier to move. But this makes it very easy to overdo it. I tend to advise doing 50 per cent less than what you think you can do – so if you think you can manage twenty minutes, try ten and see how you feel immediately after and for the next two to three days. As with cycling and walking, if that feels ok and you can repeat it twice or three times with no negative outcome, start to slowly increase what you are doing. It is advisable to rest in between lengths, especially when just starting out, gradually reducing the length of time you rest as your stamina improves.

Hydrotherapy

Hydrotherapy is exercises done in a warm pool (often between 33 and 36°C) and usually led be a physiotherapist or movement specialist. Being in water supports your weight, which helps to take the load off your joints, while the warmth can soothe pain and improve circulation, so increasing comfort levels during exercise. However, for those who struggle with heat intolerance or sensitivities, exercising in such a warm pool might be challenging.

Cold-water swimming

Cold-water swimming has become popular in recent years. It can be done in any outdoor pool, from cold water to ice-cold water (below 5°C). Several studies have shown health benefits for cold-water swimming, but it can come with some risks, too, especially due to the initial shock factor of the cold (in the first three minutes) and potential health risk to those with certain cardiovascular conditions. Prolonged immersion (more than thirty minutes) in water below 1°C can lead to hypothermia and death. Supervision is advised and a gradual, progressive-acclimatisation approach to swimming in cold water.

Anaerobic activity

Anaerobic activity is short, fast, high-intensity exercises that use a different energy system from aerobic exercise. This could include things like sprinting, heavy-weight training, spin class, jumping, etc.

This system typically uses glucose in the muscles to generate energy, rather than oxygen and can only be sustained for short bursts of time (approximately 90 to 120 seconds). To use our anaerobic systems, we typically have to be pushing our heart rates to 80–90 per cent of the maximum and it can lead to more muscle aches, as it creates lactic acid as a by-product. Generally, with autoimmune conditions, although we know exercise can help to reduce inflammation, pushing *too hard* can cause it to increase, potentially leading to more pain and fatigue. For this reason, I use the anaerobic threshold theory (see p. 205 in Chapter 11) to guide clients. Over time, we find we can manipulate the energy systems we use with how efficient we are at using them and many clients can build their capacity to cope with anaerobic exercise.

Now that you have an idea about different types of exercise, you can make a plan of what you think you will enjoy doing and ways to start. The next chapter is focused on strength exercises that will help you to build a strong foundation and support your joints through movement. These are great starting points for your strength regime and will see you through any form of exercise you have chosen from this chapter.

Measuring exertion levels

I encourage my clients to monitor their heart rate or use the Borg Rating of Perceived Exertion scale (RPE) – or use both and compare their findings.

Heart rate

Your heart rate represents how fast your heart is beating and is measured in beats per minute (bpm). You can track it using your watch, a finger probe or chest-strap device. Cardio equipment like bikes and treadmills also have heart-rate monitors built in (although accuracy can vary in my experience).

It can be helpful to know your resting heart rate to start with. Ideally, check this when you have been lying down, so your body is truly at rest. You can use your heart-rate monitor or feel your pulse on your wrist and count the beats for thirty seconds, then multiply that number by two. The average resting heart rate is between 60 and 100bpm. The lower your resting heart rate, the 'fitter' you generally are.

Note: if you are on medication that alters your heart rate, you can still use your heart rate to check in, but know that it may not be a precise measure of how hard you are working, so check with your cardiologist for advice regarding heart-rate measuring and targets.

Heart-rate targets

The harder you are working, the bigger the demand on your heart to pump blood around your body, so the higher your heart rate goes.

To calculate your safe maximum heart rate, subtract your age from 220. For example, I am thirty-one, so my safe maximum heart rate is 189bpm.

Target heart rates are used as a guide to help you know how hard you should be aiming to work. They are calculated as a percentage of your maximum heart rate, so they are specific to you and your age. For example, if I want to work at 50 per cent, I would aim to get my heart rate to 94bpm. If I want to work at 85 per cent, I would aim to get my heart rate to 160. For moderate-intensity physical activity, it is suggested your heart rate should be between 64 and 76 per cent of your maximum; for vigorous-intensity activity, it should be between 77 and 93 per cent of your maximum.

Please note that heart-rate targets will vary from individual to the next. I generally work with clients using the anaerobic threshold theory (50–60 per cent of your maximum heart rate), due to the fatigue response as part of their autoimmune condition (see Chapter 11).

Borg Rating of Perceived Exertion scale (RPE)

The RPE scale is a subjective measure for you to judge how much effort you are putting in/how hard you are working. The original Borg fifteen-point RPE scale ranged from six to twenty (to correspond with a heart rate of 60–200bpm; if you were 13 on the Borg scale, you would be aiming for a heart rate of 130bpm (i.e. 13 x 10). This was then adapted into a ten-point format (CR10 category ratio) for ease of use, with 0 being lying on a bed doing nothing and 10 being your absolute max. You track how you feel based on physical markers, such as how fast your heart feels like it is beating, how breathless you are, sweating/redness and how fatigued your muscles are.

Modified CR10 scale		Borg 15-point scale
0	Rest	6
1	Very easy, minimal effort	7–9
2	Easy	10
3	Moderate, comfortable	11–12
4	Somewhat hard	13
5	Hard	14–15
6		16
7	Very hard	17
8		18
9		19
10	Maximum exertion	20

Working with both your heart rate and RPE

There is a significant link between your heart rate and RPE. However, with some chronic conditions, the body feels out of sync. Comparing your RPE to your heart rate can be useful – for example, if your heart rate is 140bpm, but you feel you are cruising at an easy 2/10 effort wise, what's causing the mismatch? Is your autonomic nervous system (the part of the nervous system that controls unconscious functions, such as breathing, heart rate, digestion) struggling to regulate? Are you really at 2/10 or are you ignoring signs your body is working at a harder level? Or maybe your heart rate is at 90bpm, but you feel you are at 6, as your legs feel heavier with each press of the pedals. Is your body more fatigued than you thought and maybe you need to do less today or slow down? Listening to your body and using all the cues available to you helps you to relearn how it responds to exertion.

8

Exercises I –
Strength movements

It is hard to give you a prescription for movement without having met you or knowing about your body. So instead, my aim is to give you the confidence to set up, adjust and progress your exercises yourself. The exercises in this chapter all include a description and illustrations, so you can see exactly what to do.

Why these exercises?

The biggest mistake people tend to make is picking exercises that are too challenging for their body to start with. We are often dealing with muscle weakness, a reduced range of movement, guarding behaviours due to pain and altered movement patterns as a result of reduced exercise and symptoms. So we need to start with movements that we can control and are pitched at an ability-appropriate level to reduce the risk of injury or increasing symptoms.

I find it works to start with single-joint exercises that are easier to control, rather than jumping straight into compound or multi-joint movements. Once you have a baseline foundation of strength and movement again, you can layer movements and start to incorporate more compound exercises or exercises specific to what you want to do. For example, lifting your arm overhead is a single-joint exercise, versus a shoulder press, which involves bending the elbow and then moving the shoulder.

The position you exercise in also makes a difference: horizontal movements tend to be lower energy as more of your body is supported. You also have more feedback (sensory input from the surface you are lying on), which is ideal when you are trying to relearn movement patterns and build your awareness or proprioception (perception or awareness of the position and movement of the body to know how to move correctly). In sitting and standing, you are moving against gravity and have less support.

I used to find the typical physiotherapy exercises or movements in pain-management groups boring and repetitive. It is often suggested that we are limited when starting to exercise, and that wriggling our toes and rolling our wrists are our only options. In fact, there is a whole spectrum of movement you can tap into, which feels good, helps make you stronger and can be tailored to work with your body. I want you to enjoy and have fun with movement, even if it starts off looking or feeling very different to exercise pre-diagnosis.

Before we get into the exercises themselves, there are a few principles around strength training you will need to be aware of.

Progressive overload

Understanding progressive overload is the first step in setting up your strength programme. It is a principle of strength training that means you gradually increase the stress placed on the neuromuscular system (the nervous system working with the muscles) to facilitate adaptive strength. For example, if you do a body-weight squat, this challenges your muscles. By slowly doing more squats, or then adding weights, you are increasing the demands and so the body adapts. There are seven key principles to progressive overload and they can be used as a guide to slowly building up exercise tolerance and working towards whatever your goal may be.

1. **Frequency** – how often you are going to do something. As discussed in previous chapters, consistency is key, so doing something, no matter how small, helps. Although strength training is recommended twice a week, you may choose to split this into shorter, more frequent sessions – say, three or five times a week.

2. **Duration** – as with frequency, how long you do something for also impacts the results. The recommendation for strength training is two thirty-minute sessions, but again, thirty minutes could, initially, be too long for you. So it may be that your sessions need to start off at ten minutes and you gradually add time as your stamina improves.

3. **Repetitions** – the number of times you do an exercise. There are different guidelines for this, depending on your specific goal. A high number of reps (fifteen plus) at a light load (body weight only or using light weights) is helpful for building endurance, whereas low reps (one to five) with a higher load (using heavier weights) are helpful for significant increases in power and strength. It is likely you'll want to work on hypertrophy (increasing muscle mass – which means building muscle size and strength) which uses moderate loads (medium weights) with eight to twelve reps. A set is a group of repetitions, and you can do anywhere from one set to five.

4. **Rest** – involves both rest time between sets and between sessions. Rest in between sets can vary again, depending on your strength goal. For clients who struggle with fatigue or heart-rate regulation, longer rests can be beneficial. Rests between sessions are also required in order to allow time for your muscles to recover. It is helpful to have at least two rest days a week from exercise. Someone who is just starting to add in strength work may plan up to three days of rest in between sessions to allow full recovery and assess any impact.

5. **Intensity** – this is about how much effort is required to complete the exercise. Generally, the more we gently stress our tissues, the more we strengthen them and encourage growth. You can increase the load through changing your exercise position and by adding in resistance in the way of bands and weights. As your body adapts to the load, you can then increase it. It's important to start at a load you know and trust your body can handle – in most cases we start with just body-weight exercises (no added resistance).

6. **Tempo** – the speed at which you move your body also changes the load going through your muscles. Slowing down a movement or adding a hold can make it feel more challenging without adding any extra weight. It can also add variety, which is helpful for the nervous system.

7. **Variety** – you can modify exercises so that you still target the same muscle groups but in different ways. This is a balancing act, as you need to do the same thing consistently to notice improvements, but not so much that you, your

body and brain no longer find it fun or a challenge. Tweaking the exercises and mixing things up can help you to keep progressing and enjoying movement.

Strong foundations

Our bodies are constantly compensating and adapting to all that life throws at them, and living with autoimmune conditions means they often have to adapt more than others', due to procedures, operations, medical tubes, ostomies, insulin pumps and so on. Sometimes, however, these adaptions aren't helpful in the long term, and can lead to more dysfunction, pain and limitations. Then we need to relearn how to effectively move again, starting with the basics.

We want to start by rebuilding our foundations, or as I like to think of them, our 'tin-can' muscles. Our core muscles act like a cylinder around our abdominal contents, in between our ribs and pelvis. They create stability by drawing in from all four sides of the body to create intra-abdominal pressure. Exactly like a tin can around its contents. We need a strong tin can to help stabilise and provide us with support, so we can use our upper and lower bodies effectively. If our tin can isn't working in any one direction, it affects how the whole body functions.

We have our lid, aka the diaphragm, which sits at the base of our ribcage and is vital for breathing. The front of our can is made up of a muscle called transverse abdominis (TVA) – this is typically called our 'core' although lots of names for it float around the fitness world, including our deep abdominals, our powerhouse, our centre. The TVA wraps around our bodies like a corset and sits beneath three other layers of abdominal muscles (rectus abdominis, aka our 'six pack' and internal and external obliques). At the base of our tin can is our pelvic floor, which supports our pelvic organs and is vital for bladder and bowel function. And lastly, our back muscles (such as multifidus) provide support to the spine to hold us upright. We need our tin can to work as a whole, as when we move, the intra-abdominal pressure constantly changes. Normally, these muscles should work automatically, like every other muscle in the body, and the brain is constantly communicating and recruiting muscles when we need them. However, with pain and dysfunction it can be helpful to bring our awareness back to these muscles to stop others trying to take over and overcompensate. We want to bring our awareness back to building a strong foundation with our tin-can muscles before we start to layer on more dynamic movements.

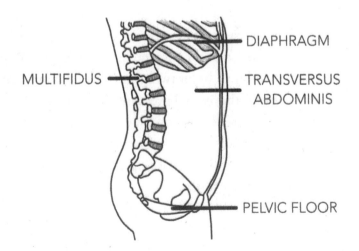

BEFORE YOU START

Here's a quick guide to some terminology and concepts to help you when you get started with movement and exercise:

Repetition (rep) = one completion of an exercise (for example, one bicep curl = 1 rep, 10 bicep curls = 10 reps)

Set = a series of repetitions performed in a row (for example, 2 sets of 10 reps)

Rest = an interval of time between sets to allow the muscles to recover, typically from 30 seconds to 2 minutes, but it can be longer

Regression = a way to make a movement easier or to adapt it

Progression = a way to make a movement harder, by changing the position or adding in resistance

Neutral spine = the term used to describe where the pelvis and lower back are not tipped forwards and backwards but comfortably in the middle; it depends on each individual what this looks and feels like for them

Breathing = there are cues for breathing to help use your breath to slow the movements down, or to use the exhale for the more challenging part of the movement and use your 'tin can' muscles effectively (see p. 95); if it feels hard to get the breathing right, just focus on not holding your breath and breathing through the movements

Breathwork

Learning how to breathe effectively is key. When we have experienced pain or trauma we can sometimes 'forget' or struggle to take deeper breaths. Not only is our diaphragm an important component of our trunk (tin-can muscles), helping us both to stabilise and allow movement, our breath also communicates a sense of safety to the brain. Deep, slow breaths activate the parasympathetic nervous system, cueing the body to feel calmer and be in a more relaxed state.

Start by noticing your normal breath. Notice where you feel it the most – the nose, throat, upper chest, ribcage or belly. Is your normal breath slow or fast? Does it feel easy or effortful? Do your inhale and exhale feel the same length? Do you feel a restriction anywhere? Once you have brought your awareness to all this, we are going to try to actively change it using two breath techniques.

DIAPHRAGMATIC BREATH

Known as deep or belly breathing, this is where you actively try to use your diaphragm as you breathe, encouraging fuller, deeper breaths.

- **Start:** any position, although you may find it easier to practise in lying or supported sitting initially. Place both hands on your lower belly or, alternatively, place one hand on your chest and one on your lower belly.

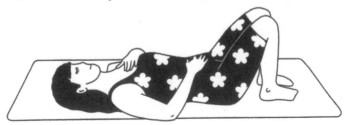

- **Movement:** inhale through the nose and try to feel your belly lifting your hands up; exhale through the nose and feel your belly soften and relax under your hands.

- **Watch points:** check you are not forcing it by using your other stomach muscles to brace and push your stomach out. Watch that you are keeping your upper chest relaxed (use the hand on your chest to feel this).

LATERAL BREATH

This breath also uses your diaphragm, but it focuses more on creating space through your lower ribcage, helping with thoracic mobility and enabling you to maximise the use of your trunk muscles as you move during the exercises.

- **Start:** any position, although you may find it easier to practise in lying or supported sitting initially. Place your hands on the sides of your ribcage, where your lower ribs are.

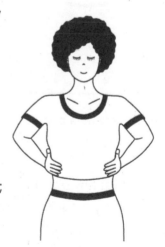

- **Movement:** inhale through the nose, trying to feel your ribs expanding out to the sides, pressing into your hands; exhale through the nose, feeling your ribs softening back to the midline.

- **Watch points:** keep your upper chest and neck relaxed. Imagine your lower ribcage has a band around it and you are trying to breathe into it.

If you are struggling to move your ribcage, try wrapping a resistance band around your lower ribs and breathe into the resistance.

Core and pelvic floor

Our core, aka transverse abdominis (TVA), works alongside our pelvic floor. Bringing your awareness to one will help with the other.

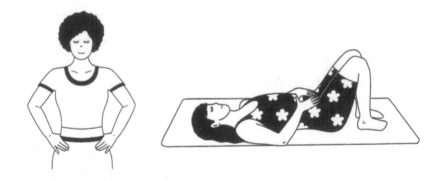

TRANSVERSE ABDOMINIS

This acts as a corset around your belly and back, supporting all your organs.

- **Start:** any position, although you may find it easier to practise in lying or supported sitting initially. Place your fingertips on your hip bones, then slide them a few centimetres down and across, into the soft area of your lower abdomen. If you laugh or cough, you should feel a muscle under your fingertips twitch or switch on.

- **Movement:** inhale, relax your stomach; exhale and gently draw in your belly button towards your spine. Try to now breathe normally whilst you hold this drawing in sensation. Imagine on a scale of 0–10 (where 0 is off and 10 is on full) – you want to work to a maximum of 1, where you are just aware of/can just feel your TVA tighten or move under your fingertips. Gradually build up the length of time you can maintain this for, until it becomes something you do not need to think about.

- **Watch points:** keep your face, legs and neck all relaxed. You should be able to keep breathing, talking and moving. If you can't, you are probably trying to grip too much. You're not aiming for a rigid, gripping of your TVA. Focus on rebuilding your awareness of it without tensing up everything else, too.

PELVIC FLOOR

This acts as a sling, supporting all the pelvic organs, while also allowing the bladder and bowel to function.

- **Start:** same position as above with your fingers down and inwards from your hip bones. You cannot feel your pelvic floor externally; however, as it contracts, you will feel your TVA switch on, too, as they work together.

- **Movement:** inhale, relax; exhale and draw your pelvic floor up and forwards. Imagine you are squeezing from your back passage all the way to the front, as if you are trying to avoid passing wind or going to the toilet. Practise contracting and relaxing quickly up to 10 times, then try contracting and holding. You want to aim to hold for up to 10 seconds, but you may need to build up to this. Then take a big inhale and feel the sensation of your pelvic floor fully relaxing when you have finished.

- **Watch points:** try to keep the rest of your body relaxed and don't hold your breath! Do not practise this while actually on the toilet.

PELVIC-FLOOR RELAXATION

Many people have pelvic-floor tension in that they are unable to fully relax and let go of the pelvic floor. You want to ensure you are letting go of tension between the exercises and allowing it to fully relax, so you can contract and relax your pelvic floor through its full range. It would be like doing a bicep exercise by bending your elbow and then never letting it fully straighten to allow your bicep a chance to relax. Think sniff, flop and drop, as follows:

- **Start:** lying, as above.

- **Movement:** inhale through the nose, as if you are doing a big a sniff. As you fill your lungs with air, imagine your belly 'flops' and your pelvic floor 'drops' down. Exhale to maintain this relaxed sensation, then repeat 2–3 times.

- **Watch points:** try to feel the 'sniff, flop, drop' all on the inhale; don't try to bear down through the exhale. You can imagine your pelvic floor is a lift, and with each inhale, as you soften, the lift moves down a level.

PELVIC TILT

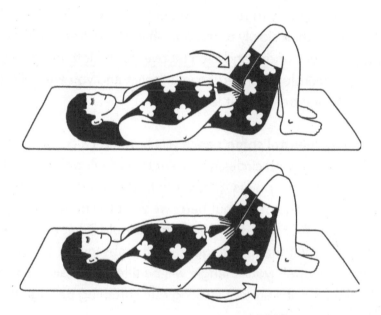

- **Start:** lying on your back, feet hip-width distance apart, knees bent, tracking over your middle two toes. Hands can be in a triangle shape over your pelvis, palms on hip bones and fingertips on your pubic bone.

- **Movement:** inhale to prepare, exhale, start to tilt your pelvis backwards, as if you are trying to gently melt the lower back into your mat or bed. Inhale to soften through the front of the hips and start to tilt the pelvis forwards, peeling your back away from the bed or mat.

- **Watch points:** try to keep your glutes and inner thighs relaxed; don't grip and tighten – find softness. The rest of the body will move a little, but this movement is minimal. Start with a really small movement and focus on its control and quality.

- **Progression:** try to take it into pelvic circles, tilting the pelvis forwards, then slowly to the right-hand side. Keep rolling back to tuck under and then tilt over to the left. Imagine you have a marble balanced on your pelvis and you are rolling it in a circle, not letting it fall off.

- **Finding 'neutral spine':** once you have had a go forwards and back or with circles, you want to try to find the middle between these points. Often, our bodies like to be in one extreme or the other, but here, we want to find the happy medium. Your palms and fingertips should be at the same level, in a flat triangle, fingers and thumbs in line. (If you are not in 'neutral', your triangle will be tilted.) You also want to watch your ribs are not sticking out, softening through the back of the ribcage.

CHIN TUCK

The chin tuck helps to build awareness and strength in the deep neck flexors. These act in a similar way to the core (TVA) and are very important for stabilising the head and neck and reducing the forward head posture commonly associated with neck pain and headaches.

- **Start:** lying on your back or sitting or standing (if sitting or standing, it can be helpful to be against a wall). Rest the palm of your hand on your nose.

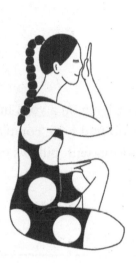 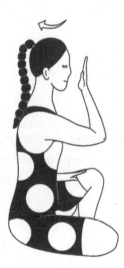

- **Movement:** inhale to prepare, then exhale and start to pull your nose away from your hand, by creating length through the back of your neck. Breathe while you hold this position, starting with three breaths (so you're not holding your breath) and building up the number of breaths you can hold it for. Then soften and relax.

- **Watch points:** you should feel the front of your deep neck muscles (deep neck flexors) switch on, but the rest of your shoulder and chest muscles should be soft. Watch you do not overtuck and strain these muscles. You want to focus on creating length through the back of the neck without dipping the chin to the chest.

- **Progression:** it is often easier to start in lying as you have the feedback from the surface you are lying on. Practising in upright positions like sitting or standing can be more challenging.

Horizontal exercises

These exercises can be done in bed or lying on a yoga mat – wherever you feel most comfortable. If you find lying completely flat a challenge, try a supported lying position with pillows or a bolster to support your spine, neck and head.

KNEE OPENING

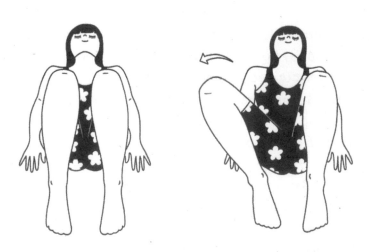

- **Start:** lying on your back, feet hip-width distance apart, knees bent, in line with your middle two toes, aware of your core and pelvis position, arms resting down by your sides.

- **Movement:** inhale to prepare, then exhale and start to float your knee out to one side, keeping your foot in contact with the ground and keeping the other knee still. Inhale and return the knee back to the start position. Repeat on the other side.

- **Watch points:** try to keep your pelvis still and not rocking or swaying from one side to the other. Imagine a glass of water on each hip bone that you don't want to spill. Keep the movement small to start with, focusing on the quality of movement.

- **Regression:** you can start by repeating on one leg at a time for all reps, before swapping.

- **Progression:** to make it harder, try adding in arm openings (see p. 116) with opposite arm and opposite knee; or try both sides at the same time for an extra challenge. You can also try adding a resistance band around your mid-thighs and pressing out into it.

THIGH SQUEEZE

- **Start:** lying on your back, feet hip-width distance apart, knees bent, tracking over your middle two toes and arms resting down by your sides. Place a small rolled-up towel or cushion between your thighs.

- **Movement:** inhale to prepare, exhale gently and press into the towel or cushion, squeezing the thighs together. Breathe to hold the squeeze for 1–5 breaths. Then relax.

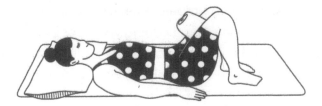

- **Watch points:** try to keep the rest of your body relaxed; try not to hold your breath.

- **Progression:** you can do a combination of slow, long holds and quick pulses. You could also use a small Pilates ball between your knees and press into it for more of a challenge.

LEG SLIDE

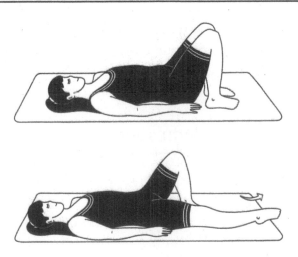

- **Start:** lying on your back, feet hip-width distance apart, knees bent, tracking over your middle two toes, aware of your core and pelvis, arms resting down by your sides.

- **Movement:** inhale to prepare, exhale to slide your foot away from you, aiming to fully straighten your leg. Inhale to slide the foot back into the start position. Imagine there is a glass of water on each hip bone, and you are trying to avoid spillages.

- **Watch points:** try to keep the imaginary glasses of water on each hip bone still. Imagine your hip, knee and ankle are all on the same track, staying in line.

- **Regression:** if you find it challenging, you can start with a small range of movement, not taking your leg all the way to straight. If you are on a non-slip surface, like your bed or a non-slip mat, wearing a sock and putting your foot on a bin bag can help to reduce the friction.

- **Progression:** try to add the opposite arm or even try raising both arms overhead as your leg slides away from you and bring them back down by your sides as the leg slides back in.

KNEE EXTENSION (AND OPTIONAL LIFT)

- **Start:** lying on your back, with a rolled-up towel or a cushion under one knee (the other leg can be straight or with your knee bent, depending on comfort), aware of your core and pelvis, arms resting down by your sides.

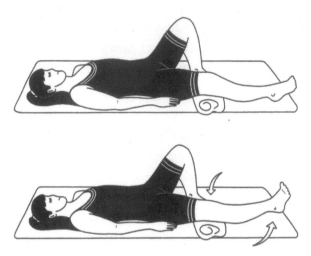

- **Movement:** inhale to prepare, exhale to squash the back of your knee into the towel or cushion, then raise your leg. Inhale to lower your leg and relax back to the start position. Exhale to repeat on the same leg.

- **Watch points:** the towel or cushion will stop you from hyperextending your knee. Watch as you lift your leg off the cushion or towel that you maintain that knee position. Imagine you are pulling your kneecap up towards you.

- **Progression:** you can add an ankle weight to make your leg heavier, aim to lift your leg higher or try the movement without the feedback/assistance of the towel or cushion.

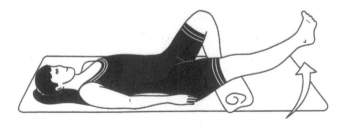

HIP LIFT TO BRIDGE

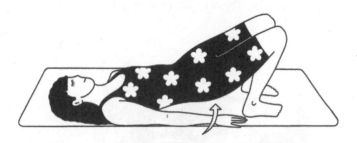

- **Start:** lying flat on your back, feet hip-width distance apart, knees bent, tracking over your middle two toes, aware of your core and pelvis, arms resting down by your sides. This is often more comfortable for your neck without a pillow.

- **Movement:** inhale to prepare, exhale to start to roll your pelvis and lower back up off the mat. Inhale to hold here. If you want to progress to a full bridge, keep rolling up, peeling off one vertebra at a time, until you are resting on your shoulder blades. Inhale to hold, exhale to start to roll back down with control, reversing the movement, lowering bone by bone.

- **Watch points:** don't focus on how high your hip lift or bridge is. Instead, focus on how long you can make your spine. Imagine someone is pulling your knees towards your toes and see how much space you can create as you go up and down.

- **Progression:** try a cushion or pillow between your knees (same as knee squeeze) and apply a gentle squeeze as you lift and lower, adding pulses at the top for an extra bonus. You can use a resistance band (loop band or long band tied around mid-thighs) and press outwards into it, so you don't let your knees fall in. You can add in heel raises or pulses up and down. You can also try and lift one leg while in your bridge!

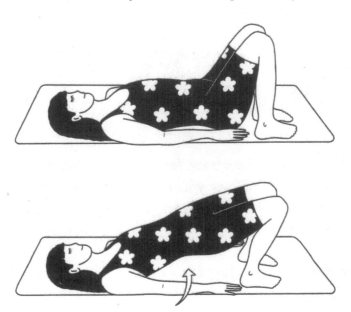

CLAM

- **Start:** lying on your side with your head supported by your bottom arm or a pillow/head block; hips and knees bent, so that your heels are in line with the rest of your spine and knees are at approximately 90°. Can you try to lengthen your top waist? Imagine you are pulling your tip hip away from your body, making your sides as long as possible, so your hip bones are stacked on top of each other. Hand can either be resting on your hip or relaxed, resting gently on the floor in front of you.

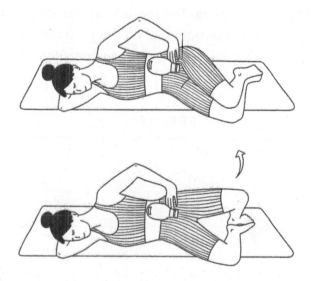

- **Movement:** inhale to prepare, exhale to lift the top knee away, keeping both heels pressed together. Inhale to lower the top knee down again with control.

- **Watch points:** don't focus on how high your knee is lifted. Focus instead on the quality of movement to try to stop your pelvis and body rocking forwards and backwards. Imagine you have a brick wall behind you, so you cannot rock backwards. Check you are using the muscles in your back-pocket region vs overusing the hip flexors (front of the hip), adjusting your foot position if needed. Relax your upper body, especially your face, jaw and neck.

- **Progression:** you can add a cushion or pillow between your knees and apply a gentle squeeze as you lower your leg down. Slow down the movement, counting to 3 as you lift or lower your knee. Add pulses at the top for an extra bonus. Add a resistance band (loop band or long band tied around mid-thighs) for an extra challenge. Or try 'floating clam', where you try to raise both feel off the ground, keeping the feet still, as if they are balanced on an imaginary stool

LATERAL LEG LIFT

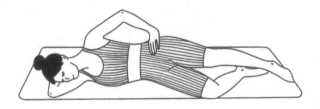

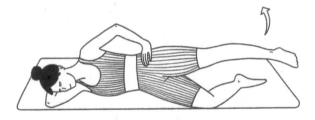

- **Start:** lying on your side, head supported with your bottom arm or a pillow/head block. Your bottom leg has a slight bend in the knee and your top leg is out straight. Imagine you are pulling your top hip away from your body, making your sides as long as possible, so your hip bones are stacked on top of each other. Your upper hand can either be resting on your hip or relaxed, resting gently on the floor in front of you.

- **Movement:** inhale to prepare, exhale to lift the top leg, so that it is in line with your top hip. Inhale to lower the leg down again with control.

- **Watch points:** don't focus on how high your leg is lifted. Focus instead on the quality of movement to try to stop your pelvis and body rocking forwards and backwards. Imagine you have a glass of water balanced on your top hip and you don't want to spill it. Watch that your top foot does not start to creep forwards; keep it in line with the rest of your spine. Relax your upper body.

- **Progression:** add pulses at the top for an additional bonus, use a resistance band (loop band or long band tied around mid-thighs) or ankle weights for an extra challenge.

ARM MARCH

- **Start:** lying flat on your back, feet hip-width distance apart, knees bent, tracking over your middle two toes, aware of your core and pelvis, arms resting down by your sides. Try a pillow or head block for support if you prefer.

- **Movement:** inhale to prepare, exhale to float both arms up towards the ceiling. Inhale to pause to find space across the collarbones. Exhale to find heaviness through the back of your shoulder blades. Inhale to check your elbows are not locked. Exhale to take one arm overhead and one by your side; inhale to draw both arms back towards the ceiling. Exhale to repeat with the opposite arm going overhead.

- **Watch points:** only take your arm overhead as far as you have 'active' control – meaning your muscles are switched on and supporting the shoulder joint. Check your ribs and

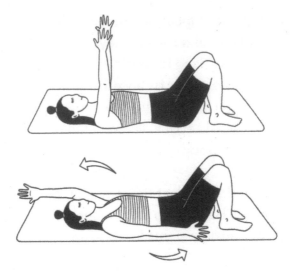

pelvis – did they move as your arm went overhead? Can you try to minimise the amount your ribs lift and press up to the ceiling?

- **Progression:** you can speed up this movement by taking away the pause, with both hands meeting at the ceiling – just breathe freely as your arms float up and down. You can also try a double-arm raise, lifting both arms overhead together and both down by your sides. Or hold a light weight or wear a wrist weight to make it harder.

ARM OPENING

- **Start:** lying flat on your back, feet hip-width distance apart, knees bent, tracking over your middle two toes. Float both arms up to the ceiling, thinking heavy shoulder blades, so that they feel like they are sinking into the surface you are lying on.

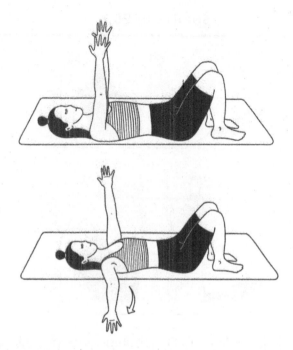

- **Movement:** inhale to prepare, exhale to open up one arm to the side, keeping the other arm still. Inhale to slowly draw the arm back to the start position. Repeat with the opposite arm.

- **Watch points:** only take your arm as far to the side as feels comfortable. Try to control the speed, keeping it the same as you open the arm and as you lift it again. Watch that you are not locking out your elbow.

- **Progression:** take both arms out at the same time and bring them in at the same time. You can also combine this movement with knee opening, trying each arm with the opposite leg, or even the same arm and the same leg for an extra challenge.

SUPINE PRESS

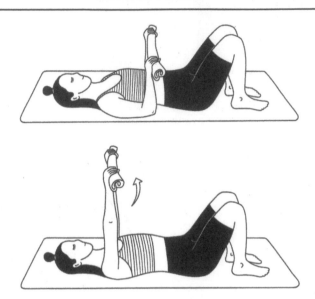

- **Start:** lying flat on your back, feet hip-width distance apart, knees bent, tracking over your middle two toes. Hold a rolled-up towel in both hands, upper arms resting on the ground and elbows bent at 90°.

- **Movement:** inhale to prepare, exhale to press the towel away from your body, up towards the ceiling. Keep a neutral wrist grip (wrists not bending forwards or back) and a light pull on the towel throughout, like you are trying to gently pull it apart. Inhale to slowly bend the elbows and lower the towel back to the start position.

- **Watch points:** keep the shoulder blades heavy throughout the movement. Watch as you press the towel up that the shoulders do not lift forwards, too. Think wide, smiley collarbones to keep your chest open.

- **Progression:** once you feel comfortable with the press, you can add lifting your arms overhead, too – only taking them as far as you can control and feels comfortable. If it feels easy with the towel, add a resistance band (either loop or long band tied). You can also progress to holding free weights with the same movement.

TRICEP DOUBLE ARM (AKA SKULL CRUSHER)

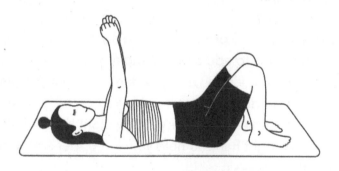

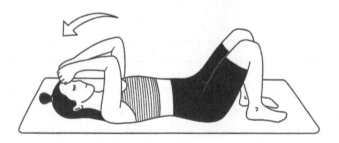

- **Start:** lying flat on your back, feet hip-width distance apart, knees bent, tracking over your middle two toes. Hold a light weight between both hands – this could be a tin can, bottle of water (with varying levels of water) or a dumbbell – with arms straight up to the ceiling.

119

- **Movement:** inhale to prepare, exhale to bend the elbows, so the weight comes down towards your forehead. Inhale to straighten your elbows, so the weight moves back to the start position.

- **Watch points:** move slowly, lifting and lowering the weight with control, making sure you don't bang your head with the weight or drop it! Keep your shoulder blades heavy on the mat, collarbones wide and check your wrists are in neutral (not bending forwards or back). Check your elbows aren't going too wide.

- **Progression:** both a progression and a way to make the exercise easier is to add a loop band around your upper arms to help guide the elbows, so they don't stick out. Progress your weight gradually to get heavier. You can also do a single-arm tricep exercise – hold the weight in your left hand, and use your right hand to hold your left upper arm to help support the elbow's position.

BICEP CURL IN LYING

- **Start:** lying flat on your back, feet hip-width distance apart, knees bent, tracking over your middle two toes. Have your arms down by your sides, with no weight or a light weight in one hand – this could be a tin can, bottle of water (with varying levels of water) or a dumbbell.

- **Movement:** inhale to prepare, then exhale to bend the elbow, so your hand lifts up towards your shoulder. Inhale to straighten your elbow, so the weight moves back to the start position.

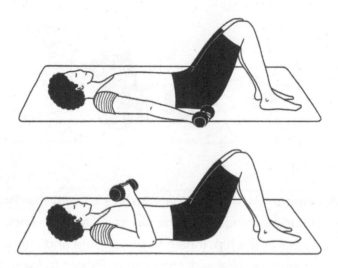

- **Watch points:** move slowly, as you lift and lower the weight. Try to maintain the same speed up and down. Keep your shoulder blades and backs of your upper arms heavy on the mat, collarbones wide and check your wrists are in neutral (not bending forwards or back).

- **Progression:** hold the weight palm facing the ceiling, as shown, or turn your wrist, so that your palm faces in towards your body and complete the movement this way. Gradually progress the weight you use and try doing one arm at a time or both arms simultaneously.

TOE TAPS

- **Start:** lying flat on your back, feet hip-width distance apart, knees bent, tracking over your middle two toes and arms resting by your sides.

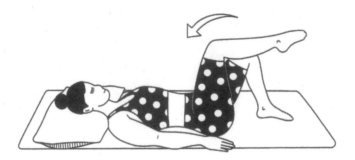

- **Movement:** inhale to prepare, exhale to float one leg up to tabletop position, with the hip at 90° and the knee, too, stacked over the hip. Inhale to pause here and check your shin bone is parallel with the ceiling. Exhale to lower the leg, maintaining the 90° knee position to tap the toe on to the surface you are lying on. Inhale to float the leg back to tabletop. Repeat on the same leg.

- **Watch points:** watch that you maintain the leg position; it should feel like your leg is moving from the hip, rather than just bending and moving the knee. Keep your foot active, with your toes pointed, but if that is not comfortable, you can flex the toes. Try to keep an even pressure through the back of the pelvis, not tilting to the side of the leg you are lifting.

- **Progression:** alternate your legs, moving one and then the other to challenge the pelvis. You can add an arm march (see p. 115), lifting the opposite arm and leg. You can then try to 'scissor' the legs – as one leg taps down, the other floats up straight away.

PRONE ARM LIFTS – 'V LIFT'

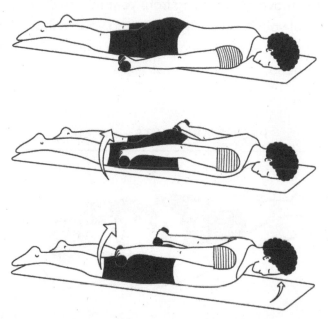

- **Start:** lying on your stomach, with your pubic bone heavy into the mat and your forehead pressing into the surface you are lying on, looking directly down. If this is uncomfortable, fold a small towel and place it under your head for support. You can start with nothing in your hands, but you have the option to add light weights (tin can, dumbbell, etc.). Keep your arms by your sides, palms facing down.

- **Movement:** inhale to prepare, keep the head where it is and lift the shoulders and the arms to hover just off the mat/bed. Inhale to hold. Exhale to gently lower. If this feels ok and you have been doing your deep neck flexor exercises (see chin tuck, p. 104), you have the option to also lift the neck and head, still looking directly down.

- **Watch points:** keep the back of the neck long. Don't let your gaze move up or hinge through the neck in either variation. Feel the movement coming from your mid-back and the middle of your shoulder blades. Keep your tailbone long – so you have a beautifully long spine from your coccyx all the way to your head.

PRONE ARM LIFTS – 'W LIFT'

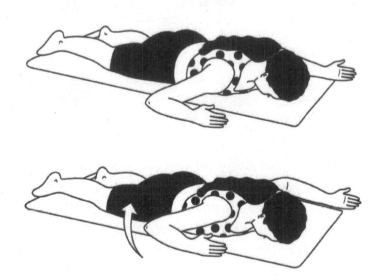

This is the same as the previous exercise, but this time your arms should be in a 'W' shape – elbows bent, and in line with your shoulders, and wrists and hands in line with your elbows, framing either side of your head. This is more challenging than having your arms in a low 'V' position. There's an option to lift your head up with this exercise. You can also extend your arms out to the sides, so they are in a 'T' position.

PRONE LEG LIFTS

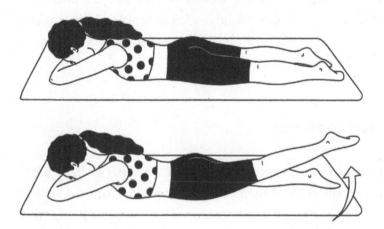

- **Start:** lying on your stomach, with your pubic bone heavy into the mat or bed, your hands are one on top of the other and your forehead is resting on top (or you can place a folded small towel or a cushion under your head for support).

- **Movement:** inhale to prepare, then exhale to lift up one leg just off the mat/bed. Inhale to slowly lower. Repeat on the same leg.

- **Watch points:** keep your tailbone long and try to stop your back from hinging, so that you have a beautifully long spine from your coccyx all the way to your head. Do not worry about how high your leg lifts. Try not to tip your pelvis from one side or the other as you lift the leg.

- **Progression:** move on to lifting alternate legs. You can also try lifting both legs at the same time. Try a resistance band looped around mid-thighs or wear ankle weights to add more load to this movement. You can combine the upper-body movements of the V or W lift (see pp. 123 and 124) while lifting one of your legs – for example, right arm and left leg, right arm and right leg, both arms and right leg or both arms and both legs all together.

Seated exercises

You can do these exercises sitting in a chair (with or without a back), on the edge of the bed, in a wheelchair or on a sofa. If you sit away from any back support, up tall on your sit bones (the bony bits of your bottom), you will use your trunk muscles more than if you lean back. Just changing the way you sit you can change the intensity of these exercises.

SEATED HEEL RAISES

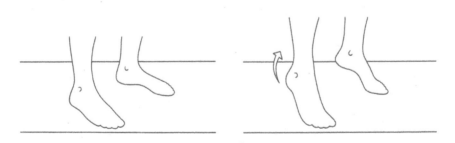

- **Start:** on a chair or the edge of a bed or sofa, sitting high on your sit bones with a long spine. Keep both feet in contact with the ground, arms resting on your lap or your hips.

- **Movement:** inhale to prepare, exhale to lift the heel of one foot. Inhale to lower. Exhale to lift the heel of the other foot. Inhale to lower.

- **Watch points:** think about your foot as having three points, like a triangle – your big toe, little toe and heel should all be pressing into the ground. Think of this triangle shape when you both lift and lower your heel – the heel should be in the centre of the two points of your toes.

- **Progression:** try lifting both heels at the same time. You can put a tennis ball or soft Pilates ball between your heels as you lift them up together, pressing into the ball.

KNEE EXTENSION

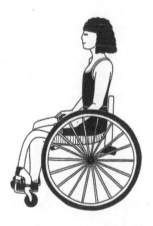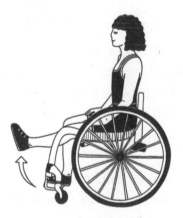

- **Start:** on a chair or the edge of a bed or sofa, sitting high on your sit bones with a long spine. Keep both feet in contact with the ground, arms resting on your lap or your hips.

- **Movement:** inhale to prepare, exhale to straighten your knee. Keep your toes active (flexed towards you, if possible). Inhale to bend the knee, lowering the foot down.

- **Watch points:** don't lock the knee by hyperextending the knee joint. Try to keep the other leg still, with the foot firmly planted on the floor. Try not to rock to the side as you do this. Keep the foot you are lifting active throughout.

- **Progression:** try a band around your lower leg and tie it to the chair for resistance or wear an ankle weight. If you tend to hyperextend the knee and lock the joint, you can put a rolled-up towel under the leg you are working (like the knee extension on page 109) to provide more feedback, so you don't lock it.

KNEE MARCHES

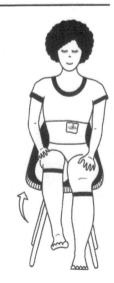

- **Start:** on a chair or the edge of a bed or sofa, sitting high on your sit bones with a long spine. Keep both feet in contact with the ground, arms resting on your lap or your hips.

- **Movement:** inhale to prepare, exhale to draw one knee up towards you, lifting the foot. Inhale to lower the foot back down, then exhale to lift the other knee and continue.

- **Watch points:** try to keep your pelvis still, not hitching or tipping to one side then the other. Try to control the movement as you lower your foot back to the floor.

- **Progression:** try a band around your mid-thighs for resistance or an ankle weight on your ankle to increase the load.

WAITER

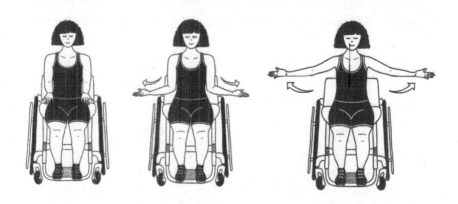

- **Start:** on a chair or the edge of a bed or sofa, sitting high on your sit bones with a long spine. Keep both your feet in contact with the ground. Bend your elbows at 90°, tucked in by your sides, palms facing up.

- **Movement:** inhale to prepare, then exhale to rotate your shoulders, taking your hands out to the sides with elbows staying tucked into your body. (You then have the option to straighten the arms out to the sides, keeping the hands lower than your shoulders.) Inhale to rotate the shoulders back in, bending the elbows, and return your arms back to the start position.

- **Watch points:** check that as you do the movement your shoulders don't move up to your ears and keep your chest wide and the back of your neck long. Watch that you don't force the movement; keep it gentle and only rotate the shoulders outwards as far as you can control and feels comfortable.

- **Progression:** try a resistance band or light weights for more resistance. You can also add some extension pulses: keep your arms in the position with hands rotated away from the body and straighten and bend the elbows for a bonus set of pulses.

SEATED ROW

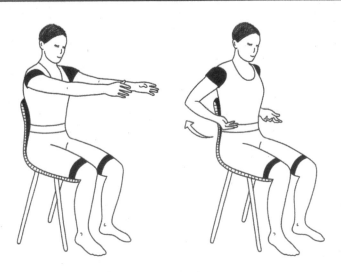

- **Start:** on a chair or the edge of a bed or sofa, sitting high on your sit bones with a long spine. Keep both feet in contact with the ground and reach both arms out in front of you, palms facing each other.

- **Movement:** inhale to prepare, exhale, bend your elbows and move them back, so your hands come in line with the side of your ribcage. Inhale to release your arms back to the start position.

- **Watch points:** check that as you do the movement your shoulders aren't moving up to your ears, keep your chest wide (to stop your shoulders dropping forwards as the arms return) and the back of your neck long. Watch that your elbows do not move out to the sides; keep them close to your body.

- **Progression:** try a resistance band or light weights for more resistance to the movement. You can also do the movement one arm at a time, adding in some gentle rotation as you pull the elbow back, twisting your upper body (while keeping your lower body still and facing forwards). Try this rotation with or without a band, too.

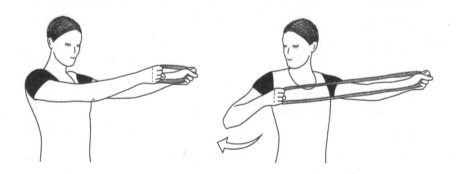

SHOULDER ABDUCTION

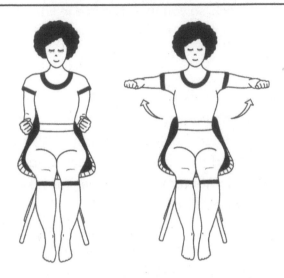

- **Start:** on a chair or the edge of a bed or sofa, sitting high on your sit bones with a long spine. Keep both feet in contact with the ground and start with your elbows bent at 90°, tucked in by your sides, palms facing each other.

- **Movement:** inhale to prepare, and exhale to lift your elbows out to the sides, so they move to be in line with your shoulders. Inhale to lower the elbows back down.

- **Watch points:** keep your elbows at 90° the whole way through the movement. Keep your chest wide and the back of your neck long. Imagine you have balloons under your armpits that inflate as you lift your arms up, and then you press the air out of them as your arms lower.

- **Progression:** try light weights for more resistance to the movement. You can have your arms out straight, so your hands are in line with your shoulders to make the movement harder – starting with your arms by your sides and lifting the whole arm up.

BICEP CURLS

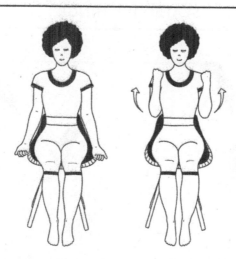

- **Start:** on a chair or the edge of a bed or sofa, sit high on your sit bones with a long spine. Keep both feet in contact with the ground and start with your arms straight down by your sides, palms facing forwards.

- **Movement:** inhale to prepare, then exhale to bend the elbows up towards the front of your shoulders. Inhale to straighten the elbows, lowering your hands back down by your sides.

- **Watch points:** check that as you do the movement, nothing else is moving. Keep your collarbones wide to prevent your shoulders moving forwards and your wrists in line with the rest of the arm.

- **Progression:** try a resistance band tied under your foot or the chair or light weights for more resistance to the movement. You can change the position of your hands to a 'hammer curl' by turning your palms to face inwards, as if you are holding a drink.

SEATED HIP HINGE

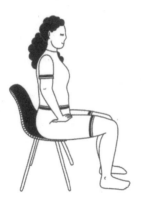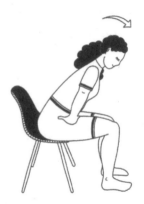

- **Start:** on a chair or the edge of a bed or sofa, sitting high on your sit bones with a long spine. Keep both feet in contact with the ground and your hands on your hip bones.

- **Movement:** inhale to prepare. Exhale to slowly soften at the front of your hips and fold forwards. Inhale, finding length through your spine and exhale to return to the starting position.

- **Watch points:** check that you are not rounding your back as you move forwards. Imagine you have a metre rule strapped to your back, and as you tip forwards you have to keep your spine long. Keep your neck in line with your spine, too, trying not to look up or down.

- **Progression:** try moving your hands to the back of your head to add more load to the movement. You can also do this exercise kneeling and standing.

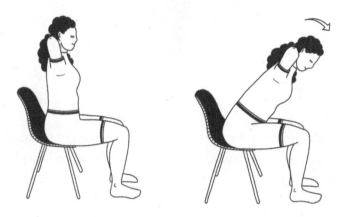

All fours

Being on all fours can be difficult, but it is a great way to challenge stability and develop strength. There are lots of options in this position, which we will now cover. Building up strong foundations in this position first is key to being able to manage other exercises on all fours.

FINDING ALL FOURS

- **Start:** on your hands and knees, with your hands under your shoulders and knees under your hips, spread your fingers like you are both trying to grip the mat but also push it away at the same time. Feel like you are pressing your shoulder blades and mid-spine up to the ceiling. Look just in front of your hands to lengthen the back of your neck. Think about the tops

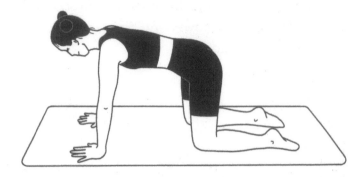

of your ears pointing forwards, rather than down or up to the ceiling. And think of drawing your lower belly up to lengthen your lower back. Press the tops of your feet into the mat.

- **Movement:** breathe and try to hold this position for 2–3 breaths and then rest. Once you feel more comfortable finding and holding this, try to breathe with some gentle sways from side to side. You could then add some soft rocking, forwards and backwards. Keep your spine long, then inhale and draw back to the start position.

- **Watch points:** watch that your elbows do not lock/hyperextend. Make sure your hips are stacked over your knees (our knees like to creep forwards).

- **Regression:** if you experience wrist pain in this position, focus on the way you set up and slowly build up to however long you can hold it for. If this still feels too much, you can always come on to your fists or use a rolled-up towel under the palms of your hands to give you more space for your wrists. You can also practise weight bearing through your wrists on tables/kitchen counters/walls.

HAND TAPS

- **Start:** on all fours (see p. 135).

- **Movement:** inhale to prepare. Exhale to tap your right hand on top of the left hand and then inhale to place it back on the floor. Then exhale as you repeat with your left hand to tap it on top of the right.

- **Watch point:** try not to rock or tip from one side to the other as you lift up one arm then the other.

SUPERMAN ARM SLIDE AND LIFT

- **Start:** on all fours (see p. 135).

- **Movement:** inhale to prepare, then exhale to slide one arm forwards along the ground. Inhale to slide the arm back. There is an option here to add in an arm lift – exhale to slide the arm forwards and then lift it up, as if you are shaking someone's hand in front of you. Inhale to lower and slide back in.

- **Watch points:** don't let your shoulder blades or upper back dip. Try not to let your body sway from one side to the other – see if you can keep an imaginary tray of drinks on your back steady. Keep looking directly down.

- **Regression:** if taking your arm forwards feels uncomfortable, try sliding your hand out to the side, to the edge of your mat. You can then also try to lift your arm to the side.

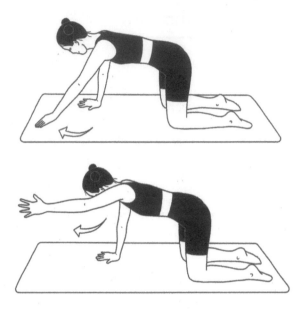

- **Progression:** try lifting your arm straight up without doing the slide first. You can hold a weight in your hand or wear a wrist weight. Try a yoga block or small Pilates ball on your lower back to provide feedback and see how much you can challenge yourself to keep your body still. You can also add taps, just lifting and lowering the arm before returning back to all fours.

SUPERMAN LEG SLIDE AND LIFT

- **Start:** on all fours (see p. 135).

- **Movement:** inhale to prepare, exhale to slide one leg backwards along the ground. Inhale to slide the leg back in to the start position. There is an option here to lift the leg, too: exhale to slide the leg backwards and then lift it off the floor, aiming for hip height. Inhale to lower and slide back in.

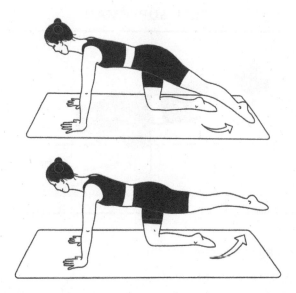

- **Watch points:** don't let your shoulder blades or lower back dip. Try not to let your body sway from one side to the other – see if you can keep an imaginary tray of drinks on your back steady. Keep looking directly down.

- **Regression:** if you struggle to not sway, make sure you stay on the same leg for full repetitions before switching to the other side.

- **Progression:** try alternating your legs. You can start to lift your leg straight up behind you without doing the slide first. You can wear an ankle weight or put a yoga block or small Pilates ball on your lower back to provide feedback and see how much you can challenge yourself to keep your body still. You can also add taps, lifting and lowering the leg before returning back to all fours.

FULL SUPERMAN

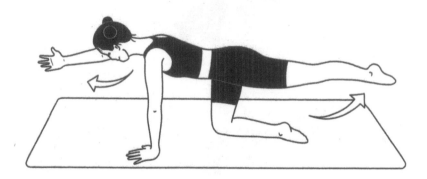

- **Start:** on all fours (see p. 135).

- **Movement:** inhale to prepare, exhale to slide one arm and the opposite leg away from you. Inhale to slide the arm and leg back. There is an option here to add in an arm and leg lift: exhale to slide the arm and leg away, then lift both off the ground. Inhale to lower and slide back in.

- **Watch points:** don't let your shoulder blades or upper back dip. Try not to let your body sway from one side to the other – see if you can keep an imaginary tray of drinks on your back steady. Keep looking directly down.

- **Progression:** try lifting your limbs straight up without doing the slide first. You can hold a weight in your hand or wear an ankle weight or put a yoga block or small Pilates ball on your lower back to provide feedback and see how much you can challenge yourself to keep your body still. Once the arm and leg are lifted, you can then tap them down to the mat and lift back up again. See how long you can keep both arm and leg lifted.

KNEE HOVER TO PLANK

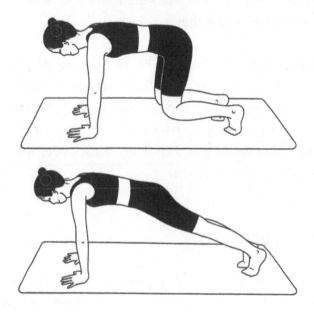

- **Start:** on all fours (see p. 135), with your toes tucked underneath you.

- **Movement:** inhale to prepare, exhale to press into your hands and toes and hover the knees just off the mat. Breathe normally as you hold, then exhale to lower. Full-plank variation: step back one leg at a time, until you are in a long, diagonal line.

- **Watch points:** don't let your shoulder blades or upper back dip. Watch you do not lock out your elbows. Keep looking directly down. If in plank, keep your pelvis in line with the rest of your spine.

- **Regression:** if lifting up your knees feels too challenging, practising holding the all-fours position will help. If your wrists struggle for full plank, you can try the forearm variation, with your elbows bent, stacked under your shoulders and palms down on the mat.

- **Progression:** with the knee hover, you can try tapping your knees down to the mat and back up again. You could add trying to combine a hand tap (see p. 137). With the plank, you can try to tap your hands, too, or tap your feet out to the sides. You could try and lift a leg or rock your whole body forwards and backwards.

Standing exercises

Standing exercises can help you to improve functional movements like getting off a bed or chair, managing stairs and picking something up off the floor. They are often more challenging, as they require you to balance, co-ordinate and control your whole body (as opposed to seated or lying exercises, where you have more support). They are, however, easily added into daily life – for example you can squeeze in some heel raises or practise standing on one leg while waiting for the kettle to boil.

HEEL RAISE

- **Start:** standing with your feet hip-width distance apart, think about spreading your toes wide. Keep your knees soft (not hyperextended) and stand tall. You can hold on to a chair or kitchen counter with two hands in front of you to start.

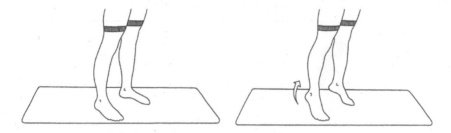

- **Movement:** inhale to prepare, then exhale to float the heels off the ground. Inhale to lower with control.

- **Watch points:** think of your foot as having three points like a triangle – your big toe and little toe and heel should all be pressing into the ground. Picture this triangle as your heel lifts and then draws a straight line as it lowers in the centre of the two points of your big and little toes. Try to stop your toes lifting off the ground, keeping them planted. Watch that your knees do not try to lock.

- **Progression:** try a tennis ball or soft Pilates ball between your ankles and try to keep it in place through your heel raise – this can help to prevent your ankles moving in and out. You can try to turn sideways, so you only hold on to your support with one hand, then a few fingers, then no support at all, to work on your balance. You can progress to doing a single-leg heel raise, lifting one foot off the ground and lifting and lowering your other heel, or try a heel raise on the edge of a step for more range, or with your weight leaning forwards.

SQUAT (WITH CHAIR)

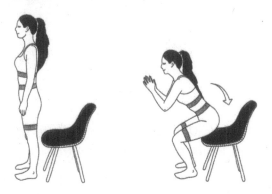

- **Start:** standing tall with your feet in a comfortable stance (hip-width distance apart or wider), knees unlocked, feet firmly planted into the ground and hands on hips or in front of you. It can be helpful to have a chair behind you to start.

- **Movement:** inhale to prepare, exhale to bend the knees and hips, sinking down into your glutes, as if you are trying to sit down. Inhale to press the ground away, straightening the hips and knees back to standing.

- **Watch points:** watch that the pelvis stays facing forwards, not twisting. Stay long through your spine, imagine you are trying to lengthen your tailbone down to the chair. Think wide sit bones as you go down and imagine them drawing back as you stand. Try to have your weight evenly balanced on both legs.

- **Regression:** you can use a chair to sit down, and then stand back up again to break up the movement. You can start by using a higher chair or stool, or a chair with cushions on it and then gradually pick lower options.

- **Progression:** you can do a squat without the chair or try sinking lower into a full squat. You can add an exercise band around your thighs to add resistance. Try a weight (dumbbell, water bottle, kettlebell) close to your chest or add a pillow or Pilates ball between your knees and add pulses at the bottom. You can hold your squat or slow it down.

HIP HINGE

- **Start:** standing tall with feet in a comfortable stance (hip-width distance apart or wider), knees with a soft bend, feet firmly planted into the ground and hands on hips.

- **Movement:** inhale to prepare, exhale to start to fold from the hips, tipping your upper body forwards. Your sit bones will move backwards but your knees and ankles stay where they are. Keep your back long and straight. Inhale to press through your feet and straighten back up to standing.

- **Watch points:** check you are not locking out your knees. Watch that your back does not curve through the movement, imagine you have a metre-long ruler taped to your back. Think about your spine being as long as possible, from the back of your neck to your tailbone. Do not let your shoulders pull forwards; try the cue 'wide collarbones' to help maintain this space.

- **Regression:** try this sitting down or kneeling. Stand one step away from a wall, and, as you hinge forwards, try to tap your sit bones against the wall for feedback.

- **Progression:** try putting your hands across your chest, or either side of your head to add more load to the movement. You can try a split stance, with one leg forward and one leg back with just the toes touching. You can then try a single-leg hinge, lifting the back leg completely off and trying to balance as you repeat the same movement. Try holding a weight (dumbbells or barbell), keeping it close to you by sliding it down the fronts of your legs.

VARIATIONS OF HIP HINGE

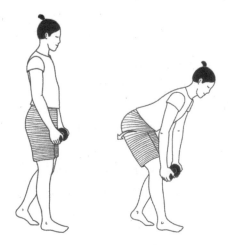

Split-stance variation; showing position to hold weight

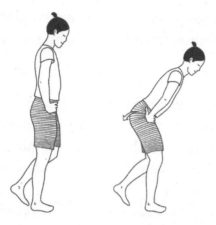

Single-leg variation with back leg lifting off

LATERAL LEG LIFT

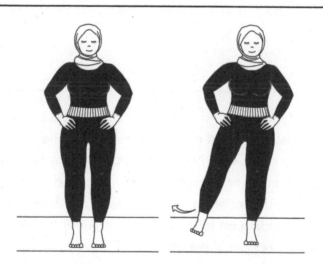

- **Start:** standing tall with feet in a comfortable stance (hip-width distance apart or wider), knees unlocked, feet firmly planted into the ground and hands on hips (or there's an option to stand sideways to a chair or countertop and hold on with the opposite hand to the leg that will lift).

147

- **Movement:** inhale to prepare, then exhale to lift one leg out to the side. Inhale to lower the leg, exhale to repeat with the same leg.

- **Watch points:** try to keep the pelvis facing forwards. Keep the leg low until you can control the movement – think quality over height to start with. Try to keep the movement slow and controlled, with the same speed going up and down.

- **Progression:** you can wear a resistance band around your mid-thigh (easier) and then around your lower leg (more challenging). You could tie a band to your ankle and loop it around something secure to pull against. Try an ankle weight or try slowing the movement down, counting to 4 up and down, or add a hold or small pulses at the top of the movement.

HIP HIKE

- **Start:** standing tall with feet in a comfortable stance (hip-width distance apart or wider). Stand with one foot on a step or a book. One knee should be unlocked and the other with a bend to accommodate standing on different surface heights with feet firmly planted. Place your hands on your hips or holding on to the back of a chair or a table with one hand for support, if needed.

- **Movement:** inhale to prepare, exhale to press off the ground and lift the leg that is on the ground. Inhale to slowly lower the leg. Exhale to repeat with the same leg.

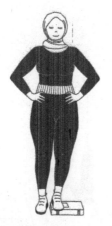 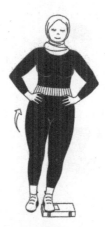

- **Watch points:** try to keep the pelvis horizontal with your hip bones in line as you lift the leg off the ground. Try to keep both hip bones facing forwards and the hip, knee and ankle in a straight line. See if you can minimise how much your body leans sideways.

- **Regression:** start with standing on a smaller/thinner book (for safety this should be pressed against a wall, so it cannot slide away). Start with holding on and gradually reduce the amount of support you need.

- **Progression:** you can try the movement with a bigger step or a stack of books or add ankle weights.

BACKWARD TAP

- **Start:** standing tall, facing a step or a thick book/stacked books, with feet firmly planted in a comfortable stance (hip-width distance apart or wider), knees unlocked and hands on hips. Step one foot on to the step or book to start.

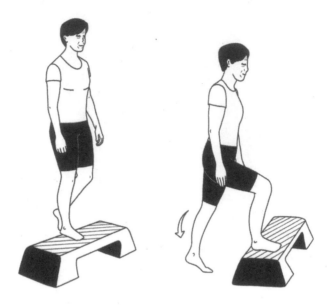

- **Movement:** inhale to prepare, exhale to step up, straightening the hip and knee of the leg on the step. Inhale to tap the back foot down with control before exhaling to repeat.

- **Watch points:** try to keep the pelvis horizontal with your hip bones in line as you lift the leg off the ground. Try to keep both hip bones facing forwards and the hip, knee and ankle in a straight line.

- **Regression:** start with standing on a smaller book (for safety, press it against a wall, so it cannot slide away). Start with holding on and gradually reduce the amount of support you need.

- **Progression:** try the movement with a bigger step. Or you can add ankle weights. You can slow down the lowering of the leg back to the ground to a count of 3.

WALL PUSH-UP

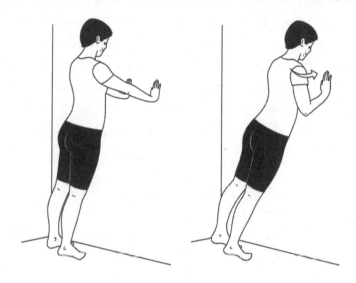

- **Start:** standing next to a wall, placing your hands on the wall, shoulder-width apart and fingers spread wide. Find width across your collarbones and keep your body in a straight line.

- **Movement:** inhale to prepare. Exhale to bend the elbows and lower your chest towards the wall; inhale to straighten your arms and push away from it.

- **Watch points:** try to keep your elbows tucked in. Watch your neck position, keeping the back of your neck long and trying not to stick your chin forwards. Keep your body in a straight line – imagine you are a plank of wood.

- **Regression:** start by standing really close to the wall, so you are upright. This reduces the load through your arms.

- **Progression:** gradually step back further from the wall, increasing the angle of your body and how much weight you load through your arms. Or enlarge the angle further by progressing the movement to a kitchen counter and increasingly lower surfaces, until you can be horizontal on your mat. You can adjust your hand and elbow position from narrow (as shown) to wider, so elbows are out to the sides. You can slow down your tempo, counting to 3 as you lower.

LINE BALANCE

- **Start:** standing tall with feet in a comfortable stance.

- **Movement:** inhale to prepare, then exhale to step one foot in front of the other, as if you are on a tightrope. Breathe to hold for as long as you can. Then swap, so the other foot is in front.

- **Watch points:** try to keep the toes pressing into the ground. Keep breathing – often, we try to hold our breath when balancing, but your body needs your diaphragm to help with stability. Keep your gaze softly focused on something ahead of you.

- **Regression:** keep your feet at hip-width distance and step one foot forwards, so you have a wider base of support. You can then steadily make your stance narrower. You can hold on to a support and then gradually reduce how much you are holding on, from one hand, to two fingers to letting go.

- **Progression:** try to move your arms forwards, up and sideways to challenge your balance. You can try to throw and catch a ball, either to yourself or someone else or you can try to close your eyes (be careful and make sure you have someone with you or are standing next to something for support in case you need it).

SINGLE-LEG BALANCE

- **Start:** standing tall with feet in a comfortable stance, hands on hips or out to the sides of your body.

- **Movement:** inhale to prepare, exhale to shift your weight on to one leg and lift the other leg just off the ground. Breathe to hold and then swap to the other side.

- **Watch points:** try to keep your toes pressed into the ground. Keep breathing – often, we try to hold our breath when balancing, but your body needs your diaphragm to help with stability. Keep your gaze softly focused on something ahead of you.

- **Regression:** you can hold on to a support and then gradually reduce this, until you can let go. Aim to hold the balance for a short time at first, building up slowly.

- **Progression:** try to move your arms forwards, up and sideways to challenge your balance. Or try to throw and catch a ball, either to yourself or someone else. You can try to close your eyes (be careful and make sure you have someone with you or are standing next to something for support in case you need it).

TOE TAPS

- **Start:** standing tall with feet in a comfortable stance, soft knees and toes spread wide.

- **Movement:** inhale to prepare and exhale to shift your weight on to your static leg and come on to tiptoes of the leg you are about to move. Breathe, as you then tap the other leg forwards, then to the side and then behind you.

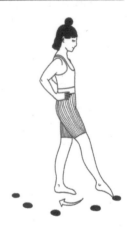

- **Watch points:** try to keep your pelvis facing forwards the whole time and stand up tall.

- **Regression:** you can slide your foot forwards, sideways and backwards along the ground (if your floor is not slippy, you can wear socks or fold a bin bag or plastic bag under your foot). Make sure your static leg is not standing on something slippy, though.

- **Progression:** you can add more of a bend into the static leg, so you are holding a demi-squat while moving your other foot.

9

Exercises II – Mobility movements

Mobility refers to how well you move your body through your normal range of motion. It describes your active range of movement, such as lifting your leg as high as it can go. This is compared to flexibility, which is how well you can move passively – if someone lifts your leg for you, for example. Mobility is a combination of flexibility, strength and stability. You need stability in some parts of the body in order to allow movement elsewhere.

Mobility movements are dynamic and are therefore a great way to warm up your body ready for exercise. They are also great in isolation. You can do mobility movements on a rest day to move your body without the intensity of strength or cardiovascular exercise. I also like doing them as a way to wind down for bed or to help me wake my body up in the morning, especially if I have woken up with stiff lupus joints.

Static stretching vs mobility

Static stretching is when you hold a certain position for at least fifteen to ninety seconds. This helps to lengthen muscles, so improving flexibility. But it only has a temporary effect on the tissues, so unless you sit in the splits all day, you will lose the benefits. We used to think static stretching before exercise would help to prevent injury, but research has shown it makes no difference. Some people find stretching helpful when muscles feel tight and painful, and it can be a useful tool for the short term. But longer term, it is better to work on your mobility, focusing on your strength and stability to help improve your range of movement.

We have a protective mechanism called the stretch reflex that prevents overstretching and injury to the soft tissues. When your muscle spindles (stretch receptors in your muscles) are stretched, they send a message via the spinal cord which immediately sends an impulse back to contract the muscle to stop it overstretching. Living with pain, we know our central nervous system is already on 'high alert' in trying to keep us safe (see Chapter 12). This can mean the nervous system is very sensitive, so if we stretch the tissues too much, it can lead to more pain and tightness afterwards – even if it feels good in the moment. It is also worth mentioning that sometimes the 'tightness' we feel isn't from muscles that are short – they may feel tight from being overworked. Therefore, you can stretch them all you want, but it never improves. This is when strengthening the muscles is more effective than stretching at helping with that 'tight' feeling.

Gentle static stretches can desensitise the nervous system's protective mechanism, but your body has to feel safe. This is why I haven't included any static stretches in this book as I feel they need to be carefully implemented with chronic pain, if used at all. I much prefer mobility movements and generally focus on normalising movement patterns and maximising the range of movement you have. This is what we are going to focus on next.

Bed mobility

These exercises are all done in lying, which can be on your bed or on your mat (or even lying on your sofa, if it is long enough). I regularly do these movements in my pyjamas and always feel better afterwards.

FOOT PEDAL

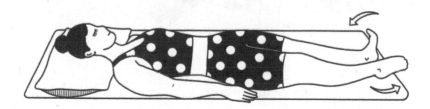

- **Start:** lying down with both legs out straight (if this is uncomfortable, you can place a rolled-up towel or pillow under your knees).

- **Movement:** inhale to prepare, then exhale to flex one foot, drawing the toes up towards your body at the same time as pointing the toes on the other foot, as if trying to reach the bed. Repeat the other way around.

- **Watch points:** try to keep your feet in line with your ankles and knees. Watch your feet to check they are not pulling to one side. Only move as much as feels comfortable. Keep the toes active throughout.

- **Regression:** you can do one foot at a time.

- **Progression:** try speeding this up. You can then add some side-to-side movements – imagine you are drawing a horizontal line with your toes – and then try ankle circles.

BOOK OPENING

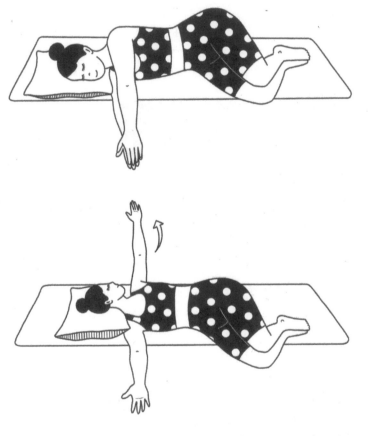

- **Start:** lying on your side with your head supported with a pillow/head block. Your knees can be bent at whatever angle feels comfortable and both arms outstretched in front of you, hands together.

- **Movement:** inhale to prepare, then exhale to lift the top arm up towards the ceiling. Once your arm is line with the rest of your body, start to rotate your torso, turning your chest towards the ceiling, too. Keep rotating and bringing your arm back behind you, as far as feels comfortable without letting your legs or pelvis follow. Inhale to hold, breathing into the side of your body. Exhale to slowly bring the arm back to the ceiling and close your book with hands reconnecting.

- **Watch points:** try to keep your legs heavy and stop your hips moving, too. Imagine your hips have two headlights on the front and stay pointing ahead of you. Watch as you bring your arm back; keep your inner upper arm within your gaze (if you can't see it, you may be overstretching your shoulder).

- **Regression:** you can try this same movement with your top arm bent, hand behind the back of your head. This time the movement is led with your elbow.

SIDE TO SIDE

- **Start:** lying on your back. There is an option to have your head supported with a pillow/head block and your knees should be bent. Bring your knees and ankles together. Have your arms slightly wider than your body in a low 'V position' with palms pressing into the floor.

- **Movement:** inhale to prepare, then exhale to start to peel your knees over to the left-hand side. Your pelvis can move but keep your shoulder blades anchored into the bed. Once

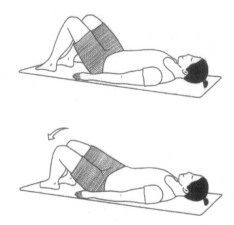

you are as rotated as far as feels comfortable, inhale to hold. Exhale from your centre, starting to draw your knees back to the middle to the start position. Inhale at the top and exhale, taking your knees over to repeat on the right side.

- **Watch points:** do not let your shoulder blades lift up. Try to breathe into the side of the ribcage to create as much space through your side as possible.

- **Regression:** you can put a pillow between your knees and gently squeeze to help control the movement.

- **Progression:** you can bring both legs into double tabletop (hips and knees at 90°, with your feet in the air), slowly bringing your legs over to one side in the same way.

DYNAMIC HAMSTRING

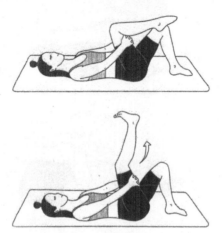

- **Start:** lying on your back, with the option to have your head supported with a pillow/head block. Have your knees bent up, then take the back of one of your legs into your hands, fingers interlaced behind your thigh.

- **Movement:** inhale to prepare, then exhale to straighten the knee as much as you can. Inhale to then flex the foot, pulling the toes towards you. Exhale to then release the foot and bend the knee again.

- **Watch points:** only straight the leg as much as feels comfortable – a slight stretch is ok but you don't want to overstretch. Keep your upper body relaxed, using pillows for support if needed underneath your head and neck. Keep your tailbone pressing into the bed.

- **Option:** you can try this with a strap or resistance band around your foot.

KNEE HUG

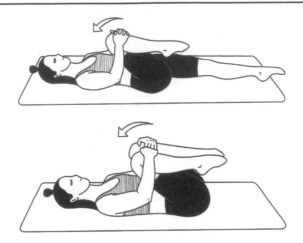

- **Start:** lying on your back (you can have your head supported with a pillow/head block), with both legs out straight.

- **Movement:** inhale to prepare, then exhale to slide one leg towards you, bending the knee and using your hands to hug the knee towards your chest. Breathe to hold. (A double-leg variation is to hug both knees at the same time.)

- **Watch points:** only bend the knee and hip towards you as much as feels comfortable; do not force it with your hands. Keep your upper body relaxed, using cushions for support, if needed, underneath your head and neck. Keep your tailbone pressed into the bed.

- **Option:** you can add an ankle circle or foot pedal while hugging your knee/knees. You can gently rotate your hip with a single-knee hug or rock from side to side with a double-knee hug.

GLUTE ROTATION

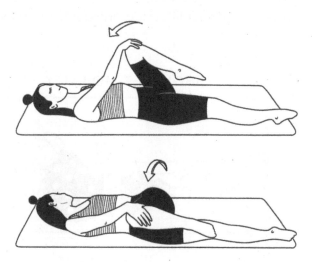

- **Start:** lying on your back (you can have your head supported with a pillow/head block), with both legs out straight and your hands by your sides, but in a wide, low 'V' shape.

- **Movement:** inhale to prepare, then exhale to slide your right leg towards you, bending the knee and using your left hand to hug the knee towards your chest. Inhale to hold, then exhale to start to guide your right knee over to your left-hand side (with an option to twist and look over your right shoulder at the same time). Your right arm is there for support, to counterbalance, and your left arm to support your lifted leg. Breathe to hold, then exhale to return back to the centre.

- **Watch points:** only rotate as much as is comfortable; do not force it with your hands. Keep your shoulder blades anchored into the surface you are lying on. Your pelvis can move, but your shoulders should stay still.

- **Option:** you can use pillows or a cushion under your knee for support if the pressure to hold it is too great. Equally, you can rest the foot of your lifted leg on your bottom leg.

SHOULDER MOBILITY

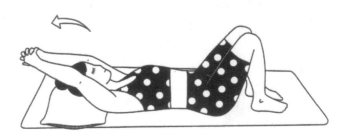

- **Start:** lying on your back (you can have your head supported with a pillow/head block), with your legs in a comfortable position.

- **Movement:** inhale to interlace your fingers together, then exhale to slowly raise your hands up to the ceiling and gently overhead, as far as you can. Inhale to feel your hands reaching away from your body, making your spine as long as possible. Exhale to lower your arms back down.

- **Watch points:** only take the hands above your head as far as you can control the movement – think active range, not passive (see p. 155). Try to keep the back of your ribcage heavy into the mat to stop your ribs from flaring.

- **Option:** you can make this into an arm circle by releasing the hands when they are overhead and sweeping them out to the sides of your body, until they are back down by your sides.

Seated mobility

These exercises can be adapted to sitting on your bed, sofa, wheelchair, mat, etc. If you spend a lot of time at your desk, they are also good to get your thoracic spine, shoulders and neck moving.

NECK MOVEMENTS

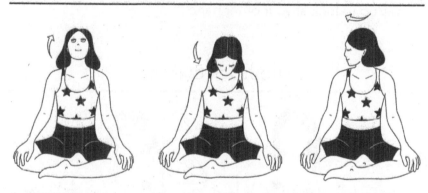

- **Start:** sitting on your mat (you can kneel or sit cross-legged, with an option to sit on a cushion to open up through the hips), on a chair or in a wheelchair. Think wide collarbones, arms relaxed, resting on your legs, with a slight chin tuck to lengthen the back of your neck.

- **Movement:** inhale to prepare, then exhale to look down, flexing your neck. Inhale back to centre. Exhale to look up to where the wall meets the ceiling, inhale back to centre. Exhale to look over your left shoulder, inhale back to centre. Exhale to look over your right shoulder, inhale back to centre.

- **Watch points:** only move the neck as far as is comfortable; do not force it. Move in a slow and controlled manner, using your breath. Keep your collarbones wide and sit up nice and tall to lengthen your spine. Do not hold it as a static stretch – instead, focus on the quality of movement.

- **Option:** try adding in a lateral tilt by drawing your right ear to your right shoulder and then your left ear to your left shoulder. You can then draw a smiley face with your nose, looking at one of your hands, then a line down and all the way up to look at your other hand.

SHOULDER CIRCLES

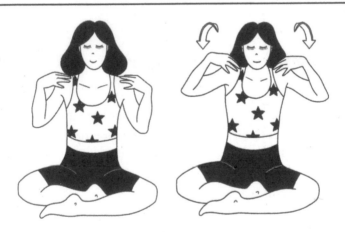

- **Start:** sitting on your mat (you can kneel or sit cross-legged, with an option to sit on a cushion to open up through the hips), on a chair or in a wheelchair. Think wide collarbones, with your hands on your shoulders.

- **Movement:** inhale to prepare, exhale to start to draw small circles with your elbows backwards. You should feel your shoulders start to move, too. Breathe as you start to make the circles bigger, encouraging a bigger circle at your shoulders. You can change direction circling forwards, too.

- **Watch points:** only move the shoulders as much as is comfortable. Try to keep the rest of your body still.

- **Option:** if having your hands on your shoulders feels uncomfortable, relax them on your lap and draw circles with your shoulders. You can make your circles as big or as small as you want.

MERMAID

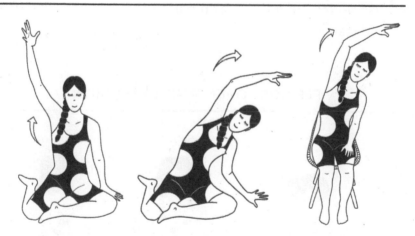

- **Start:** sitting on a chair or the end of a bed or in a wheelchair, sit high on your sit bones (the bony bits of your bottom) with a long spine. Keep both feet in contact with the ground, arms resting on your lap.

- **Movement:** inhale to lift the right arm up to the ceiling, then exhale to take the arm to the right and bend your spine over to follow it, creating a curve with your body. Inhale to return the spine and arm back to the centre and lower the arm.

- **Watch points:** try to keep even weight through both your sit bones. See if you can make an even curve through your whole spine as you bend to the side. Watch you don't move forwards or backwards, and that your ribcage doesn't twist. Keep your collarbones and hip bones facing the front the whole time.

- **Option:** try this in different positions, such as sitting on your mat or in standing. You can try windmill mermaid, where you transition from one side to the other. You can also try this sitting on a gym ball to challenge your balance and stability.

FLEXION, OPEN AND EXTENSION

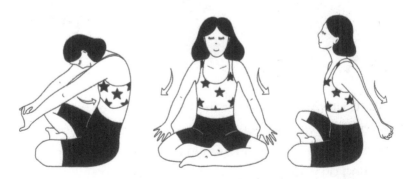

- **Start:** sitting on your mat (you can kneel or sit cross-legged, and there's an option to sit on a cushion to open up through the hips), on a chair or in a wheelchair.

- **Movement:** inhale to prepare, interlacing the fingers in front of you and turning the palms away, then exhale to gently push your hands away from your body, as you start to round your spine and drop your chin to your chest. Inhale to hold. Exhale to release your hands and send them out wide, opening through your chest. Inhale to bring your hands all the way behind you, interlacing your fingers again, palms clasped together. Exhale to draw your hands down and away, looking gently up to where the wall meets the ceiling.

- **Watch points:** only move within a range that feels comfortable; do not force it. Try to focus on the process of the movement, not just the end positions.

- **Option:** you can make this movement much smaller or bigger, depending on how it feels for you. This is similar to cat/cow (see p. 171), but in a seated position.

ROTATION

- **Start:** kneeling on your mat, sitting on a chair or in a wheelchair. Think wide collarbones, arms relaxed and resting on your legs in front of you with a long spine, all the way up to the back of your neck.

- **Movement:** inhale to prepare, then exhale to slide your right hand away towards your knee and gently rotate your upper body towards your left side, with an option to add looking over your left shoulder. Inhale to hold, then exhale to return to centre, sliding the arm back.

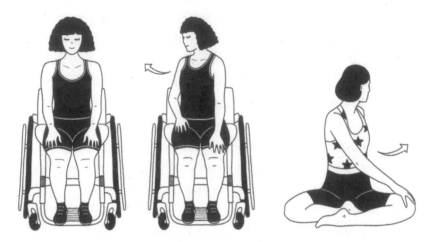

- **Watch points:** only rotate as much as feels comfortable; do not force it. Focus on the length of the spine before you twist. Keep your hip bones facing forwards – only your upper body rotates.

- **Option:** you can play with this movement by either having your arms crossed on your chest or your hands behind the back of your head, elbows wide. You can also do this in a cross-legged position and use your arms to help you twist. Place your right hand on your left knee, your left hand behind your left hip and then rotate to your left and look over your shoulder.

All-fours mobility

All fours is another position that feels good to move in, with the added benefit of building up your tolerance for being on your hands and knees.

CAT/COW

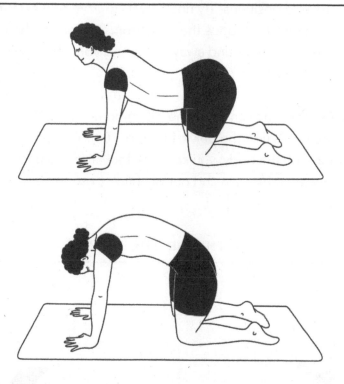

- **Start:** set up on all fours – on your hands and knees, with your hands under your shoulders and knees under your hips. Spread your fingers like you are trying to grip the mat but also push it away at the same time. Keep the back of your feet, shins and knees pressed into the mat.

- **Movement:** inhale to start to open up through the chest, lift the head and sink your belly down towards the floor in cow pose, opening up your front body. Exhale to press into your hands, tuck your tailbone and peel your back towards the ceiling, pressing the ground away from you and dropping your head down, into cat pose, opening up your back body.

- **Watch points:** focus on the movement, rather than just the end positions. Try not to just go from one extreme to the other, but notice the transition. Stay active throughout, pushing the ground away and using your strength to control the movement.

- **Option:** you can make the movement smaller, focusing on just the pelvis (like the pelvic tilt on p. 103). You can add circles through the body; you can rock forwards and backwards (like you are moving in and out of child's pose – see p. 173).

THREAD THE NEEDLE

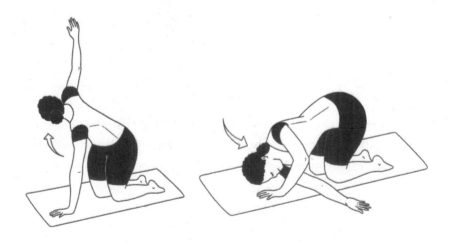

- **Start:** set up on all fours – on your hands and knees, with your hands under your shoulders and knees under your hips. Spread your fingers like you are trying to grip the mat but also push it away at the same time. Keep the back of your feet, shins and knees pressed into the mat.

- **Movement:** inhale to start lifting one arm up towards the ceiling, rotating your upper body, while keeping your pelvis facing the mat. Exhale to start to thread the raised hand under the opposite armpit and lower the same arm and shoulder down to the mat. Inhale to unwind, returning so that your arm is raised towards the ceiling.

- **Watch points:** try to keep your hip bones facing the mat; do not let them twist. Follow your raised hand with your gaze – if you can't see it, you may have taken it too far overhead, overstretching the shoulder.

- **Option:** you can bring your heels together and keep the knees wide to make a triangle base of support with the legs, which helps to stabilise your lower body as you twist. You can do the same movement with a bent arm – have one hand on the back of your head, keeping it there as you open your elbow out to the side and twist your body up to the ceiling. You can be in child's pose (the next exercise) and then thread the needle (this exercise!), if holding yourself up on all fours is a challenge.

CHILD'S POSE

- **Start:** set up on all fours – on your hands and knees, with your hands under your shoulders and knees under your hips. Spread your fingers like you are trying to grip the mat but also push it away at the same time. Keep the back of your feet, shins and knees pressed into the mat.

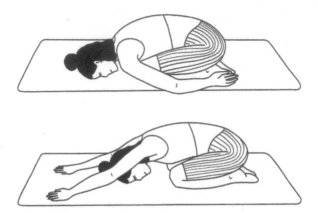

- **Movement:** inhale to start to open up through the chest, then exhale to press back, softening through the front of the hips and melting backwards until your sit bones are back, resting on your heels. There's an option to keep your arms outstretched or soften them and draw them in down by your sides.

- **Watch points:** try to have your sit bones resting on your heels (if you cannot reach your heels, use a pillow – or two or three – stacked under your sit bones and in between your heels; you can then gradually remove these).

- **Option:** you can add thread the needle (the previous exercise) by taking your right arm and sliding it under your left armpit, twisting your upper body to look under your armpit, too. You can also add a lateral stretch – if both arms are out in front, walk them over to your right-hand side, stack your left hand on top of your right and breathe into the left-hand side of the ribcage. Exhale to walk the hands back to the centre and repeat on the other side.

KNEELING TWIST

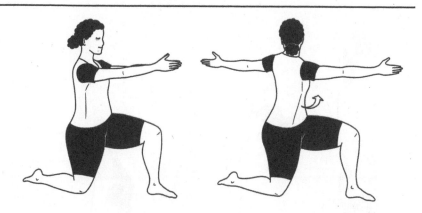

- **Start:** set up on all fours, then step one foot forwards and push yourself up, so you are in a single-kneeling position. Bring both arms up to shoulder height, pointing in front of you, palms together.

- **Movement:** with your right foot forwards, inhale to prepare, then exhale to start to open your right arm out to the right side and twist round to the right side. Inhale to hold, then exhale to rotate your upper body and arm back to centre. Inhale to pause, exhale to open the left arm out as you twist to the left side, then inhale to return to centre. Repeat with the left leg in front.

- **Watch points:** try to keep hip bones facing forwards the whole time. Only take your arm out to the side as far as you can follow it with your gaze. Try to keep your balance as you open up to both sides.

- **Option:** you can do this same movement in side lying (see book opening, p. 158).

ROLL DOWN

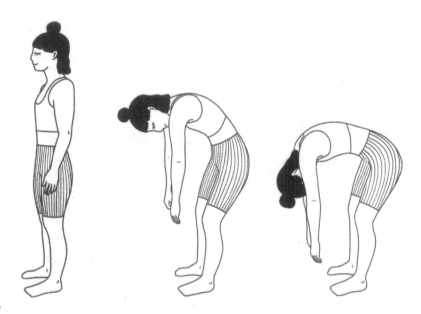

We have one standing mobility exercise (which can also be done in a seated position), and it's my favourite mobility movement for moving the spine – ideal if you have woken up feeling stiff and sore in the morning or have spent a lot of time at your desk.

- **Start:** standing tall, feet hip-width distance apart, toes spread wide, knees soft and not locked back, pelvis in neutral, ribs stacked over pelvis, shoulders wide and back of the neck long.

- **Movement:** inhale to prepare finding length through the body, then exhale to start to tuck the chin to your chest, roll through the shoulders and slowly fold yourself forwards, as if you are peeling one vertebra at a time away from an imaginary wall behind you. Lastly, let your pelvis roll forwards and let your head and arms hang. Inhale at the bottom and then exhale to start to roll up from your pelvis, restacking each vertebra one on top of the other, until your shoulders draw down your back and your head floats up last.

- **Watch points:** see how slowly you can move, really trying to feel each position as you roll down and up. Make sure you have a soft bend in the knees and deepen this if you need to, depending on your hamstring mobility. Watch that you relax your neck and don't try to hold your head up, looking forwards.

- **Option:** try this in a seated position, with legs wide, and slowly peel yourself down in between your legs. Or you can do this standing against a wall to get the feedback of slowly peeling away from the wall.

Before we go on to adapting exercise in the next chapter, here is a broad exercise plan to help you schedule in movement. I wish I could give a standard plan, but everyone's bodies and starting points are so different, so this is more of a guide that you can adapt and play around with in a way that works best for you.

Exercise plan

I recommend you start with the strong foundations (pp. 98-105) and feel comfortable with these before adding in the exercises, but what you choose to do will depend on your baseline.

To start

- Pick 1–3 foundation exercises or mobility movements as a warm-up. Do 3–6 repetitions of each.
- Pick 6 main exercises (or fewer, if this is too much; you can always start with 1!). Start with 1 set of 5–10 repetitions, aiming to build to 3 sets of 10.
- Pick 1–3 mobility exercises to cool down; do 3–10 repetitions of each.

Example exercise sessions

Warm-up (lying):	Warm-up (lying):
Breathing	Breathing
Pelvic tilt	Pelvic tilt
Shoulder mobility	Arm march

Main exercises:	**Main exercises:**
Arm opening	Leg slide
Knee opening	Toe taps
Supine press	Prone arm lifts
Knee extension	Prone leg lifts
	Hip lift to bridge
	Clam
Cool-down:	**Cool-down:**
Arm march	Book opening
Knee hug	Dynamic hamstring
Side to side	Glute rotation
Breathing	Breathing

Warm-up (sitting):	**Warm-up (standing):**
Breathing	Breathing
Pelvic tilt (sitting)	Roll down
Seated heel raises	Heel raises (standing)
Main exercises:	**Main exercises:**
Knee extension	Hip hinge (standing)
Waiter	Wall push-up
Seated hip hinge	Hip hike
Seated row	Bicep curls (seated)
Knee marches	Backward tap
Squat (with chair)	Waiter
Cool-down:	**Cool-down:**
Shoulder circles	Mermaid
Flexion, open and extension	Rotation
Kneeling twist	Cat/cow
Breathing	Breathing

Example weekly schedules

Rest days can include mobility or functional activity days.

Weekly sessions	Day 1	Day 2	Day 3	Day 4	Day 5	Day 6	Day 7
2 strength sessions	Strength	Rest	Rest	Strength	Rest	Rest	Rest
2 strength with 1 cardio	Strength	Mobility	Rest	Strength	Mobility	Rest	Cardio
3 strength sessions	Strength	Rest	Strength	Rest	Strength	Rest	Rest
3 strength sessions with 1 cardio	Strength	Rest	Strength	Rest	Strength	Rest	Cardio
2 cardio and 3 strength sessions	Cardio	Rest	Strength	Cardio	Strength	Rest	Strength

10

Adapting exercise

Yay! You have successfully added more movement into your routine. Your next challenge is to sustain it.

Hopefully, the amount you are doing is within your baseline level, so it should be manageable through small fluctuations of how you feel. However, sometimes you'll need to adapt this when your health changes more drastically or a situation arises that prevents you from keeping up your routine. In these situations, it can feel frustrating and even make you want to give up. It can feel like all that hard work, time and energy installing your schedule and building up your activity levels have been lost. Being unable to exercise can sometimes remind you of being stuck, back where you were earlier on in your health journey. Then, when you feel ready to add in movement again, it can feel like you are starting from scratch – like you've hit a snake on that snakes-and-ladders board and gone all the way back to the first square.

I have been there myself countless times, recovering from procedures, infections and hospital stays and I know it can become the biggest mental challenge. Physically starting again was ok – I knew I had to build up slowly. But mentally, it was so challenging – starting to build up my consistency and progress, only to have to stop. Again. And again. And again. So I decided I needed to change my mindset around this and think of it less as a start/stop process, but instead, a continuous one. Ongoing. Sometimes I would be doing more and sometimes less, but I wasn't stopping. I was just adjusting how much I could do.

I like to think of exercise on a dial: when things are good, we can slowly dial up the amount we do. When things are not so good, or we have busy periods, with other things going on, we dial it down. Sometimes it may be dialled down to zero movement, and that's ok, too. Sometimes exercise is a definite no, maybe stopping is appropriate medically or just what your body needs physically and mentally.

For me, this 'dial' mindset helped me to cope, both with the ups and downs, as well as with progress. The start/stop mentality often ended up with me waiting until I was 'ready' to add movement back in, whereas the continuous dial view allowed me do tiny bits here and there when I had to dial things down, and slowly add in more when I could dial it back up. It removed that big barrier of when to restart (much like the 'I'll-start-on-Monday' or 'I'll-try-again-in-the-new-year' mentalities). Plus, it meant not having bigger and longer gaps in between formal movement.

I also make sure I include all activities into what counts as movement. For example, when I am unwell, having returned home from a hospital stay, say, just walking around the house or doing a couple of domestic chores – like simply trying to wash my face, brush my teeth or get changed – requires more energy. Even walking from one room to another can wipe me out. Then, in time, I might start to add in some functional activities, like loading the dishwasher or putting on some laundry. Gradually, as I move back towards my pre-hospital baseline, these everyday tasks become easier again and I can start to do more formal movement, like walking out of the house, cycling and Pilates. It may take a week or two to reach this stage, and for some people it might feel like they are doing nothing and becoming increasingly deconditioned. However, I know that in this time, I am still moving my body and challenging it through functional activities, slowly rebuilding my strength and stamina. *All movement counts*, and it's helpful to remember this when you feel stuck and unable to do what you would typically class as 'exercise'.

Understanding your baseline in this way helps you adapt your activity levels to how your body is feeling. The rest of this chapter describes scenarios in which your baseline may change as part of living with an autoimmune condition and how I would approach handling this in terms of exercise:

1. A flare

This could be an autoimmune flare, typically classed as when your condition becomes 'active' or symptoms ramp up. A flare looks different from one person to the next, but generally, it means your body is struggling more with an increase in inflammation, which may affect specific areas (for example, joints, gut or skin) or cause more systemic symptoms (like an increase in fatigue, a sore throat, fever and so on). Normally, you can tell when your condition is flaring, but occasionally, it will be discovered in test results (such as bloods or a scan) before you notice it yourself. How you adapt will depend on how your flare is impacting you, but typically, it will cause an increase in pain, so changing how you move could help (staying in supportive positions to exercise – lying down, for example, or staying within a smaller range when moving your body). A flare will also likely increase your fatigue levels, so reducing the amount you are doing and reprioritising your functional tasks may help to keep some space for movement. If you struggle with brain fog as part of your flare, sticking to familiar and easy exercises can help to reduce the cognitive load.

2. Treatment

Following an infusion or other medical treatment, you might not feel up to your usual level of exercise. This is when the 'dial' may be turned down, with a few extra rest days. I used to have a weekly treatment and for three days afterwards, I'd be out of it and need more rest. I would try to plan my week to include more movement prior to the treatment, knowing the rest of my week would look a lot more horizontal and sedentary. Then, when I felt better again, I would prioritise movement to ensure I got back into it as soon as I could. Again, it all depends on how unwell you feel and what (if any) side effects you experience, as to whether you give yourself more rest days or try to do something on those recovery days. Movement can be a supportive tool, so maybe if you have had an IV infusion and are feeling achy in your joints, some gentle movements will feel helpful to ease the stiffness and move everything around in your system. It may be that you can still exercise or go for a walk, but at a reduced intensity – again, turning the dial down.

3. Hospital admission

For a shorter stay, if you are not feeling too unwell or sleep-deprived, I would recommend trying some movements in bed (see pp. 157–64) or even a little walk around the ward (unless you've been told by your medical team that it is not safe for you to do so). For an extended stay (perhaps weeks or months), movement becomes more important in terms of maintaining strength and function to help when you get home, and trying to keep a sense of routine, too – say, freshening up in the morning, whether that's just brushing your teeth or having a shower.

There is no need to stress about exercise, though, while you're in. I always say the real recovery starts when you are home, so anything you can do in hospital is about supporting your body as best you can and trying to reconnect with yourself and feel as human as possible.

4. Surgery/procedure

It used to be that you were advised to rest to aid recovery post-surgery, but this is quite rare now (although it does depend on what you have undergone), and getting up and walking as soon as you are medically stable is said to aid recovery. Most likely, there will be some restrictions as to what you should and shouldn't do for four to six weeks following surgery, usually related to the type of exercise or lifting, for example. This doesn't mean you cannot do anything, though, and gentle mobility movements, walking, breathwork and so on are generally allowed, but make sure you clear this with your medical team first. It's also important that you continue to check in with how you feel and how you are recovering. Everyone's timeline is different, and with chronic illness in particular, baselines can vary, so affecting when you are ready for exercise. The type of surgery and the body part affected will also impact your exercise 'dial'. For example, with an ankle procedure you may be able to adapt and move your upper body from a seated or lying position, whereas an abdominal procedure makes all movements more challenging, so it may be you can do less overall during that recovery time.

Once you have the medical all-clear to add in more exercise, don't be blinded by the green light and just go go go. Reflect back to your baseline pre-op and what you were able to do then and start with less than that. You want movement to feel easy and be able to do it consistently, slowly increasing the intensity, duration and types of exercise. It can be a challenge to know what's 'normal' post-procedure but be alert to anything that doesn't feel right to you, trust your instincts and be sure to reach out to your medical team if you have concerns. It's better to feel reassured and confident to keep going than worry or panic that something does not feel right and could be causing harm. You want your brain to get the message that movement is safe!

5. Injury

In some cases, injuries can be more common in people with chronic conditions – the body's proprioception (its sense of positioning in space) is altered due to pain, oedema (swelling) and changes to the neuromuscular system. This, combined with deconditioning, impacts strength and balance, making a roll of the ankle or tweaking the hip more likely. It is important here to recognise the difference between an acute injury and the ongoing chronic inflammatory response you are, perhaps, used to. An injury is more likely to be on one side (say, left ankle), whereas autoimmune pain is often bilateral (although one side can be worse than the other). An injury will commonly also involve an acute response that's different to your normal symptoms – maybe redness, swelling or moving differently from the other side.

Sometimes there is a clear mechanism of how an injury happened – for example, you fell down the stairs – other times it may less obvious, as it came on gradually or didn't arise from a specific event. Remember your perception will play a role here, too, based on previous beliefs around pain, your experience and the impact you think this injury will have. Pain is not always equal to the amount of tissue damage sustained.

The impact of injury on your exercise routine will depend on the type of injury and where it is. It may be that you have to modify it to reduce the load on the area you have injured – for example, seated or lying exercises with a lower-limb injury or lower-body work with an upper-body injury. You may need some time off exercise altogether to rest. In terms of the injury itself, guidance from a professional may be needed to know how to rehab it back to normal functioning. Your first goals will be to reinstate a normal range of movement in that joint and then to regain functional use, building strength and stability to prevent a similar injury happening again.

6. DOMS

Delayed onset muscle soreness (DOMS) normally starts to develop in the body twelve to twenty-four hours after exercise but can peak up to seventy-two hours after. It can sometimes be accompanied by swelling of the affected limbs, stiffness or reduced range of motion of the joint, feeling tender to touch and decreased strength. In extreme cases, elevated creatine kinase (CK) enzyme can show in the blood, signalling muscle-tissue damage and putting the kidneys at risk.

DOMS is thought to be temporary muscle damage. Exercise puts a load through the muscles, which causes microscopic damage in the muscle fibres. Over time, the muscle adapts to the damage and that's how we get stronger. This also means the severity of DOMS reduces as your body adapts to the load.

We know DOMS can be more intense with eccentric exercises than concentric. Eccentric means you are lengthening a muscle as you load it – for example, in a bicep curl, as you straighten your arm, that's an eccentric bicep muscle contraction. Concentric means you are shortening the muscle – imagine that same bicep curl as you now bend the elbow back towards you. The severity of the DOMS depends on the types of forces placed on the muscle, so if you are new to a certain activity or suddenly step up your programme a level with heavier weights, more reps/sets, etc., you are likely to experience more DOMS. One way to prevent DOMS is by progressing your programme or activity slowly. A warm-up is important but there is no evidence that this can prevent or reduce DOMS; likewise, post-exercise stretches have not been shown to help with muscle recovery and reducing muscle soreness.

DOMS generally gets better on its own in a few days. However, you may want to include rest days or lower-activity days while you are experiencing symptoms. Gentle movement may help you feel better, but again, there is no research to show this helps with recovery from DOMS. Things like ice, gentle massage and oral pain relief can help to manage the symptoms.

It's important to differentiate any muscle soreness from your usual chronic pain – usually, you can tell from the location, how it feels and the pattern or symptoms. Either way, if your pain ramps up following an exercise session, it may be that you need to reduce the intensity down for the next time, so it is more manageable.

7. Infection

As mentioned in Chapter 5, an acute illness like an infection may be a reason to not exercise. This depends on where the infection is and how much it is impacting you. A infected cut on your finger may just mean you adapt your workout not to put pressure through your hand, whereas a bladder infection with a fever and high pain may mean you have to take some rest days until your treatment has alleviated the symptoms. With anything where you have a fever or systemic signs of feeling unwell, it is important you rest. Equally, with a chest infection or symptoms below the neck you want to wait for an improvement before continuing (mobility movements or breathwork could be useful here – see pp. 155–77 and 98–100). If you do not get many infections, you may decide to dial down your exercise and rest while you recover. However, if you live with chronic infections, it may be that you decide to carry on exercising at a lower intensity or modifying, so you have a less start/stop approach to exercise.

8. **The impact of hormones**
Research has shown that there is a menstrual-cycle-related variability in the severity of pain in chronic-pain conditions. Research is limited, but a few studies have shown that pain is higher during the early follicular (during a period) and late luteal phases. In both of these, oestrogen is low, which is thought to push the body into more of an inflammatory state. This also links with how fluctuations in oestrogen, progesterone and testosterone may impact energy levels and how the body copes with exercise. It may be, therefore, that during the early follicular and late luteal phases, low-intensity exercise is favoured, compared to the late follicular, ovulation and early–mid-luteal phases, when moderate-high intensity exercise might be favoured. More research is needed in this area to better understand

how pain, energy, performance and recovery are impacted throughout the cycle.

The main thing is to adapt to how you're feeling. Some people might just want to curl up with a heat pad during a period, but if you do feel like moving, it is safe to exercise and may help to ease menstrual symptoms. You may just need to adjust the intensity. Throughout your cycle, you may notice fluctuating energy levels and pain, whereas someone else may not notice or feel that different. With so many other layers of health issues to contend with, the menstrual cycle can feel like yet another thing for the body to cope with, so give yourself compassion if you're not able to work with your cycle and find movement a challenge with hormonal changes.

There is currently little guidance around exercise in perimenopause and the menopause. We know exercise is helpful, but there is little support for navigating it. Women are more likely to suffer chronic pain than men, with the highest prevalence seen during the menopausal stage of life. There are still gaps in research as to the cause, but it is thought that along with changes affecting sleep, mood and physical activity, the change in hormone levels impacts pain sensitivity, which can exacerbate or make you more vulnerable to developing chronic-pain conditions.

9. Fun reasons

There can be multiple other reasons why you may need to adapt movement and not just for health. It could be you have an event, a weekend away, family staying or an overseas holiday. As much as aiming for consistency is important, you are also allowed time off from thinking about and doing exercise – maybe even completely. Often, you end up doing more at these times in some respects, whether through socialising or more functional movement, like exploring while away, and it becomes harder to juggle your energy balance with formal exercise, too. I try to use movement in this way to support my body to manage whatever the 'fun' thing may be. For example, if I am visiting family in the UK, I can be away for four to six weeks, which is a long time to do no exercise at all, so I may plan to fit in intentional movement when I have quieter days. However, on a short weekend away, I may focus more on rest, balancing my activity (like step counts) to ensure I do not unintentionally overdo it and then add in some mobility work before bed to help calm my nervous system.

Taking the pressure off what you think movement 'should' look like can help whenever there is a change to your normal routine, whether good or bad. While being rigid with your exercise regime can initially help to build consistency, being flexible and adapting to whatever life throws at you helps you not to fall into that all-or-nothing mindset. Remember, you can turn your dial up or down on exercise whenever you need to – just try not to leave it switched off for too long!

Exercising with fatigue

Fatigue is the most common symptom among individuals living with autoimmune conditions. Fatigue has been described by PROMIS (the Patient Reported Outcome Measurement Information System) as 'an overwhelming debilitating and sustained sense of exhaustion that decreases one's ability to carry out daily activities, including the ability to work effectively and function in family or social roles'. It is thought of as an imbalance between the energy we have available and the energy we expend.

Fatigue can be both physical and cognitive and, with no approved treatments currently to effectively treat it, it often comes down to an individual's ability to manage their energy. Fatigue is one of the hardest symptoms to push through in terms of exercise. It can often feel like our limbs are really heavy or like we're moving through wet concrete. This also affects motivation and our drive to move our bodies. When I feel fatigued, even breathing is effortful, and actively choosing to add in more movement feels like the last thing I want to be doing.

Before we talk about strategies to manage fatigue, I find it helpful to try and understand what it is and what's causing it. It is invisible, making it hard to explain to yourself, let alone others. Acute fatigue or feeling tired is a healthy adaptive response to physical and mental exertion and usually resolves with rest or sleep. Persistent or chronic fatigue, however, is often disproportionate to the activity undertaken and not resolved by rest. Part of the reason why there's no cure for fatigue is that there is still some debate over exactly what causes it.

Without getting too heavily into the science, fatigue is very much a real physical phenomenon. Research has shown that persistent fatigue has been associated with low-grade inflammation. Inflammation is something that probably everyone who lives with an autoimmune condition has in common, whether it affects one specific part of the body or is systemic. It is thought that inflammation in the body changes how we generate energy within our cells. It impacts sleep quality and how our circadian rhythm behaves. It has also been shown to impact our oxygen and nutrient supply, our metabolism, mood and motivation. All of which adds to feeling fatigued. We know that the central nervous system (brain and spinal cord) is also impacted, with changes in inflammatory mediators. This is thought to affect the way messages are relayed and could be why people with autoimmune conditions experience 'brain fog' (a term used to describe symptoms related to effortful and reduced mental functioning in areas like memory, focus and clarity). Brain fog heavily impacts my ability to find words and it has been fascinating reading back over earlier drafts of this book, as I can see when I was more fatigued when writing.

There is also research proposing that fatigue is an adaptive process to help the body conserve energy, focusing its limited supply on fighting whatever it perceives as a threat. We can all relate to this, as fatigue is a common symptom of everyday colds and viruses.

We may still come across professionals who hold that fatigue is due to becoming progressively deconditioned – that all we need do is 'pull ourselves together' and get active. But fatigue is real and persistent, and hopefully these outdated judgemental and baseless beliefs will become less prevalent over time. Research is growing all the time, with long Covid in particular having prompted more investment into this area. So there is hope that the more we learn about fatigue, the more we can help to manage it and, hopefully, have better treatment options in the future.

How can we manage fatigue?

Managing fatigue follows many of the same principles considered in earlier chapters when looking at how to introduce movement.

The nature of many autoimmune conditions is that there are periods of time with fewer symptoms and then there are flares, and fatigue is usually worse during the latter. Often, an increase in fatigue is one of the first symptoms many people notice and is therefore a sign of a flare in their condition. I think this ebb and flow in fatigue levels is inevitable, so to aim for zero fluctuation is probably unrealistic, but what can be detrimental to health and wellbeing is crashing into severe, debilitating, persistent fatigue. Finding a consistent baseline of activity that can work safely alongside our fatigue levels is hard, but it's the most important part of our movement journey.

As you'll see, there are several approaches to understanding fatigue and energy, as well as to balancing rest and activity. What works for you depends on how you like to think – whether you are more of a visual person or whether you love analysing data. Some methods can be helpful for those around you to understand fatigue and others make it easier for you to check in with your symptoms. But they all have the same underlying principles of finding safe ways for you to work with your body, so that you make progress rather than experience a wipeout.

Spoon theory

The spoon theory was created by Christine Miserandino when trying to help her friend understand what it was like to live with lupus. She grabbed a bunch of spoons and handed them to her friend and said, 'Here you go. You have lupus.' She then explained that the spoons represented the limited amount of energy she had to spend each day. Each activity had a cost, measured in spoons. For example, brushing teeth could use up one spoon, while bigger tasks, like showering or going to work, used up multiple spoons. By the end of the day, Christine's friend had only one spoon left and Christine explained that she now had to choose whether to cook, eat, clean up or get ready for bed. She described how you could borrow a spoon from the next day, but then there would be fewer left for that day. But you couldn't hoard spoons – so resting a lot one day would not mean double spoons the next. It doesn't work that way.

The spoon theory can be a helpful way to understand that everything uses energy, and that when looking at how you can work with your body, you need to factor in everything that you do. It can be a helpful way for family and friends to gain an understanding, too.

Energy budget

The energy budget is another metaphor to help track your energy, which is similar to the spoon theory. The idea is that you give yourself a budget for the day (say, £20) and each task costs you money – perhaps £2 for getting dressed or £10 for going to work. If you end up in debt from overspending your energy budget, it can take time to slowly repay that. This overlaps with my theory called the 'fun tax'.

The 'fun tax' is the increase in symptoms experienced after having some sort of 'fun'. The cycle often starts with feeling anxious prior to an activity, worrying if you will be well enough to do it or if you will have to cancel. You may worry if you can manage the whole thing and plan for different scenarios if you can't. The anxiety is rational and based on previous experience – from understanding the energy you use to push through to manage the fun and knowing that you may pay for it later with a higher level of symptoms and fatigue. The payback phase is tough – you are the one who must go through the suffering afterwards, curled up at home, alone, while others are able to go straight back into their normal everyday activities. Often, you may feel guilty about letting friends or family down if you need to cancel. Then there is the worry about whether you have made the right decision. It can also feel hard during the 'fun' activity to really enjoy yourself, due to worrying about the fun tax that will follow.

Sometimes the activity in question is so much fun that you forget to check in with yourself, ignoring early warning signs from your body that perhaps you are pushing too much, and doing more than you'd planned. Or maybe you recognise when you need to rest but choose to push through anyway. The fun-tax symptoms can hit anywhere from one to three days post-fun, so it can sometimes take a while to truly know how your body has coped. It can be really frustrating, especially if you tried hard to avoid the fun tax and stay within what you thought your body could cope with. If you chose to push, it can feel easier to accept the payback, but it still feels rubbish having to recover from a simple activity that other people wouldn't give a second thought to.

Then there is the 'loan shark' (because don't I always like to take an analogy that bit further?), encountered when you 'borrow' far more energy than you can afford, leading to a more catastrophic crash. Sometimes this can take much longer to pay back, and for some who live with ME/CFS it can lead to months or years in which their condition is exacerbated.

Activity cup

Another metaphor, and one we have already explored in Chapter 6, this is a way of looking at all the possible activity we are doing and trying to prevent the cup from 'overflowing' (see pp. 56–9).

Pacing

Pacing used to be the word I hated the most as a teenager. For me, it was boring and often meant dull days, missing out on things and hours of enforced rest. I see pacing so differently now. I find it yet another useful strategy that has changed my ability to function and increased my capacity when living with fatigue.

Pacing is described as moving or developing something at a particular rate or speed and, in the context of chronic illness, this would be a slow and steady amount in order to avoid overexertion. It is a term that is thrown around a lot but is neither very specific nor helpful, unless accompanied by an understanding of what pacing should look like *for you*, depending on your level of function, your condition/symptoms and your activity levels. So I like to think in terms of two levels of pacing: 'perfect pacing' and 'practical pacing'.

Perfect pacing, as the name suggests, is in an ideal world, when you have your whole day to yourself, completely on your terms, and can decide how best to work with your body, choosing what to do and when. You can then stack activities and rest in a way that works for you, without any extrinsic pressure. When your symptoms are very high, you may have no choice but to do perfect pacing, as without it, you are unable to function.

Practical pacing is when you try to pace yourself, but life gets in the way. Maybe your dog needs a walk, but you don't feel up to it; maybe you have to go to work for several hours more than would be ideal; maybe you have children to run around after or someone else to care for or factor in. These pressures and demands can alter how effectively you can pace. With practical pacing, you adapt depending on what your reality is on any given day.

I used to blame myself for being 'rubbish at pacing', especially in the early years of trying to juggle work and life. I'd be hard on myself for always getting it wrong, misjudging the balance and pushing too far. I then realised that being hard on myself was not helping. I instead needed to look at how I could create a more supportive balance with changes that were within my control. Pacing and modern life can feel like an impossible combination with the world being built on how productive and busy you can be. But we all deserve to work within what our bodies can cope with and just 'be' the rest of the time.

Energy envelope

This is a self-management tool designed by psychology professor and researcher of CFS Dr Leonard Jason to help with pacing and reduce symptom severity. Your energy envelope is how much you can do without exacerbating symptoms or triggering a post-exertional malaise response. It refers to a comfortable amount of energy use, where you neither overdo nor underdo it in order to maintain your activity levels.

Your envelope may be very small, without much capacity for many activities, but by staying within it you experience fewer crashes and it may lead to developing a bigger envelope. Research has shown that those who function within their energy envelope have consistently better health outcomes and quality of life than those who overspend their energy. It has a lot of similarities with pacing strategies but can be a helpful visual to work within.

Useable hours

This is one of my favourite tools. I ask my clients, 'How many useable hours do you have a day?' This means how many hours can you function? It needs to include everything you do, from personal care to food prep and meals, working or studying, medical management, household tasks, etc. The idea is that this number of hours is sustainable with your baseline symptoms – it is what you can manage without leading to a crash or flare. (It may be that you have the option to push and use eight hours a day, but if you did this every day, your fatigue or pain would worsen.) It can be helpful to assess your current baseline hours – four hours, for example – and then compare this to what you are actually using and check if there is a discrepancy. Looking at useable hours helps to give you a quick snapshot of whether you are trying to do too much each day.

Tracking fatigue levels

As we saw earlier, one of the reasons why fatigue is so hard to live with is because it can be difficult to quantify or track, as it's a feeling you often can't put into words and you cannot just choose to show your 'battery level' as a percentage. How fatigue presents can vary from person to person. They key is to understand what your baseline is. For some, their baseline may be living without fatigue or brain fog, while for others, it may be expecting some level of fatigue that remains relatively stable. In order to try to avoid that boom-and-bust pattern, you want to keep yourself around baseline, so it's useful to try to tune into what your baseline really is.

Data tracking

Thanks to technology, we now have the option to track our heart and respiratory rates, blood pressure, step count and sleep quality, and this can be super helpful or overwhelming or even lead to obsession, depending on the individual. When life is already taken up with so much health-related baggage, symptoms and medical appointments, it is understandable if you don't want to spend more time focusing on your medical data. So as with most things in life, a balanced approach is ideal. The information *can* be a helpful add-on to how you assess and work with your body. I encourage my clients, if they are able, to use this kind of data to tune into their own bodies and notice how this feels to them – for example, if their heart rate is showing as high on their smart watch, can they notice any manifestations of that within their bodies?

Benefits of data tracking

Using data can help you set boundaries for what you are doing. For example, your heart rate can guide you on how hard you are working, or your step count can help you plan your day so that you stay within what your body can cope with. Objective data can help remind you to listen to your body while it whispers – before it screams at you to stop. It can also be helpful to share that with those around you, so that they can better understand and support you with pacing. Plus, it can help your medical team, too, in providing them with more information about how your body is doing. Checking in with your data at the start of the day can be a useful way to assess where you are with your baseline – for example, resting heart rate or heart rate variability (see opposite). Lastly, using data can be motivating to note progress where otherwise it may be invisible.

Using data to manage fatigue

The table opposite shows how you can use your data to track your body's responses and adapt activity levels accordingly.

	What is it?	How to take it?	What should it be?	How can you use it?
Resting heart rate (RHR)	The number of times your heart beats per minute (bpm) at rest	Measure your pulse in beats per minute (bpm) either manually or via a device, first thing in the morning, lying down.	Between 60 and 100bpm, depending on your age. A lower resting heart rate implies better cardiovascular health – for example, an athlete's RHR may be as low as 40bpm.	Get a sense of your baseline resting heart rate – what's your average? Compare this with how you feel each day, with symptoms and energy levels. Notice if your resting heart rate is higher than normal and see if you need to adjust your activity level.
Heart rate variability (HRV)	The measure of natural variation between heartbeats. Looks at the balance of the SNS and PNS (see p. 224).	This cannot be measured manually and needs to be on a heart monitor like an electrocardiogram (ECG). Smart watches often track this, too.	A healthy HRV is 100+ milliseconds (ms). What is 'normal' varies with age and gender. Generally, a higher HRV is good and lower HRV shows dysregulation or that the body is under stress.	Looking at your HRV can help you see how 'ready' you are. A lower HRV may be a sign to take things slower and look at using tools to calm down your nervous system with habits like rest, nutrition, reducing stress, etc.

	What is it?	How to take it?	What should it be?	How can you use it?
Anaerobic threshold (AT)	The threshold measured by the heart rate (bpm) at which our bodies change the system they use to generate energy (see box opposite).	The gold standard is through lactate testing, which is not possible at home. For an estimate of your AT at 60 per cent of your maximum heart rate, use this equation: (220 - age) x 0.6 = AT	Your AT should give you a guide heart rate to stay below, give or take 5bpm.	The use of AT is to help you manage your symptoms and prevent you from experiencing post-exertional malaise. If you are still symptomatic in this range, it may be that you need to calculate it at 50 per cent of your maximum heart rate, using 0.5 in the equation.

Anaerobic threshold (AT) theory

This theory has been related to helping reduce post-exertional malaise symptoms which are seen in conditions such as ME/CFS. I have also found it a useful principle to apply to clients with autoimmune conditions who are struggling with energy crashes and symptoms post-exercise, as well as those with different forms of dysautonomia, such as PoTS (postural orthostatic tachycardia syndrome – see p. 16). The pathophysiology of post-exertional malaise is still not fully understood, but theories around metabolic abnormalities, ineffective mitochondrial energy production, nervous system abnormalities, altered immune responses and build-up of post-exercise toxins have all been considered. Based on the principle that oxidative metabolism (the chemical process in which oxygen is used to make energy from carbohydrates) is impaired, the anaerobic threshold theory advises that you keep your heart rate below a certain number (see table opposite).

WHAT ACTUALLY IS THE ANAEROBIC THRESHOLD?

Physical activity creates more demands on the body for oxygen, blood flow and nutrients and requires more energy to keep your muscles working. ATP (adenosine triphosphate) is the energy used by cells. It is made by breaking down carbohydrates (glucose), lipids (fats) and proteins. During light exercise, we typically have adequate oxygen needed to break down sugar (glucose) and fat to make our energy. Our heart rates gently increase to bring in more oxygenated blood to the muscles which is why it is often called 'aerobic activity'.

With more endurance work or when our bodies have bigger energy demands, the body cannot keep up with the oxygen needs, despite breathing more quickly and raising our heart rate further to try to pump the oxygenated blood around. Our muscles then shift to working without oxygen (anaerobically), where the body transitions to using glucose and stops breaking down fats to make energy. When we use glucose without oxygen, it creates lactic acid, which we then need to clear away, and we do so by activating our sympathetic nervous system (fight-or-flight response). Lactic acid can be responsible for fatigue and muscle soreness.

Hopefully, by now, you have gained a fuller understanding of fatigue, and have perhaps chosen a method or two that you find beneficial in helping you either to track or set boundaries around your activity levels. The next step is to understand rest.

Rest

Even though I am a huge advocate of movement, I spend a lot of my time telling people to do the opposite, helping them both to understand the types of rest and to create effective rest schedules.

Living with chronic illness, you often feel you do not have much choice when it comes to rest – you simply have to rest more. But did you know there is more to it than just resting? How you rest and when are important, too.

Resting – defined in the online Oxford Languages dictionary as 1. 'to cease work or movement in order to relax, sleep or recover strength. 2. To be placed or supported so as to stay in a specified position' – is different when living with fatigue compared to resting when you are tired. With normal tiredness, resting is used to remedy how you feel with a nap, an early night or chilling out watching TV to switch off for a bit. You would normally feel much better from a rest and can return to normal activities. With fatigue, rest is not a quick fix (you could rest for ever and still feel fatigued) – rather, it is a management tool. What is key for managing fatigue is a careful balance of rest and activity, making rest a useful strategy for pacing and balancing your energy across the day.

How to rest

Rest can look like many different things, depending on what your body needs in that moment. It doesn't have to be sleep or lying in bed. It can be physical, mental, spiritual, sensory, emotional, creative or social (the seven forms of rest, as defined by physician and researcher Dr Dalton Smith).

Physical rest can be passive, just physically being still or taking a nap/sleeping. It can also take an active form, such as mobility movements (see pp. 155–77), a gentle walk, restorative yoga and so on. After a busy day of work or something mentally taxing, sometimes filling up your social cup or doing something creative can be restful. Deciding what you find restful for different situations can be helpful. Try making a list of all the options and store it on your phone or somewhere you can easily access it. Often, in the moment, we forget what can be helpful, so this can serve as a useful reminder.

Those who say 'I can't rest' are usually the ones who need it the most. This is likely when your sympathetic nervous system (see p. 224) is so ramped up, it's like your foot is stuck on the accelerator and your body feels it cannot stop. If you then lie down and try to nap, your brain questions what you are doing – maybe by running through all the things on your to-do list, reminding you of what it perceives you *should* be doing – and you find it hard to be still; you may fidget, struggle to get comfortable and perhaps feel physical sensations, like your heart beating faster in your chest. (I often feel like I am vibrating all over when I am overtired and due a rest.) When you are in this heightened state, it is no wonder you feel unable to rest; expecting your body to immediately find the brake and slow down is unrealistic. So you need to train your body to rest – gradually help it to find the brakes by supporting the parasympathetic nervous system to take the reins moving into a 'rest-and-digest' state (see p. 224). It may be that you start with more active forms of rest, shorter rests or use tools to help you, such as visualisations or meditations. The more you teach your body how to rest, the easier it will be. It's like sleep-training a baby: there are lots of methods to choose from to get there, it will take a while and there may be tears and tantrums but, eventually, you will find rest a positive feature in your life.

When to rest

I often tell my clients the ideal time to plan to rest is before you feel you need it. We want you to rest before your body has pushed into feeling more fatigued, which usually means it has already gone into doing more than it can cope with. Also, because so many of us live with constant symptoms, we become very good at ignoring the earlier signs that our bodies need to rest and only listen when they give us no choice. For me, the signs that I am starting to need to rest are that my tailbone feels bruised, and I begin to feel frustrated that I can't find the words I want. If I can catch it in time, I can start to bring my body back to its resting state without too much trouble. When I push past this point, it takes a lot longer to do this. (To pick up the sleep-training analogy again, this is not dissimilar to trying to put an overtired baby down for a nap.) The more you push past what your body can cope with, the more you ramp up the sympathetic nervous system.

So no matter what else is happening on any given day, regardless of how busy or stressed I may feel – even if I feel better some days and don't need it in the same way as other days – I still rest. It also helps me to set boundaries with both myself and my work, friends and family. I often work in the morning and the evening, and every day, from 1–3pm, I go upstairs to rest. This is my protected time. On weekends, if we are planning an outing, we factor in my rest. I am flexible, and sometimes it may be slightly earlier or later, but I need that rest point in my day to be able to function, day in, day out.

You might find it helpful to start with a rigid rest schedule to help get you into the habit. Use the tools you would use to remind you to do other activities, like exercise, by setting alarms, writing reminders, stacking rest – for example, I have lunch and I rest after that. Be consistent with your rest and notice the difference.

How long should you rest for?

This depends on the type of rest you are choosing. It may involve taking yourself into a quiet, dark room for a more formal rest period, maybe even a nap. I usually recommend blocking out between one and a half and two hours if you are aiming for a forty-five-minute sleep, to allow for winding-down and coming-round time before and after. For those who cannot escape for this length of time, whether due to work or looking after children, I encourage micro-breaks throughout the day. This could be anything from a five-minute break up to twenty minutes. Even taking what I call a 'breath break', where you take a few deep breaths can be restful. In short, there is no ideal 'dose' of rest. It's about finding a balance that works for you – something that fits into your lifestyle and helps you support your body throughout the day.

SNEAKY RESTROOM BREAK

This is my favourite form of rest when I am out somewhere. If there is a quiet room I can go to, I will choose that; otherwise, I'll take myself off to the toilets, sit in a cubicle, on the loo (with the lid down!) and close my eyes. Focusing on my breath, I check in with myself, then I take a few slower, fuller deep breaths. I stay there for maybe five minutes, then go back to whatever event I'm attending.

This a great way to add in some restorative breaths and assess how you're doing. It's easy in a social situation to be caught up in things, running on adrenaline and not recognising your body's needs before it's too late and you have overdone it. This little hack gives you that opportunity to check in with yourself and perhaps see what you need in that moment. It helps you to connect back to yourself and calm your body down using your breath.

To nap or not to nap?

As a teenager with insomnia I was lectured about taking naps and told I was not allowed to sleep at all in the day. Sleep hygiene is definitely key when trying to manage insomnia – things like going to bed and waking up at the same time every night/morning, rules regarding screen use around bedtime and creating a good routine to help the body know it's time to sleep. However, this does not mean you should never take naps, especially when you add them in correctly.

I found if I was only getting two to three hours of sleep at night, then not napping during the day, I was operating with such a huge sleep deficit my body was running on empty. Incorporating a nap actually helped my sleep, as by the time bedtime came around, I wasn't completely overtired and in survival mode. My daily nap has also been a game changer in managing chronic migraine and helping with my overall pain levels.

Research is mixed regarding the pros and cons of napping. One study has shown that in healthy adults, frequent napping, along with napping later in the day, can impact your sleep quality with longer times to fall asleep and waking up during the night. Another study suggests excessive sleep and frequent naps can increase systemic inflammation, whereas another suggests naps can help with immune function. Many studies also show that napping can lead to improvements in cognition and may help with emotional regulation, too. A nap of sixty to ninety minutes can give you the same performance benefits as a whole night's sleep. A study looking at older adults suggested that banning all naps may not be helpful, as the benefits and the potential impact on sleep varies, depending on age and sleep requirements.

Limited studies have looked directly at naps in chronic illness. In patients with fibromyalgia, they found daytime napping for more than thirty minutes increased pain, fatigue, depression and memory difficulties, while reducing sleep quality. They also found an association between daytime naps, especially in the afternoon, and reduced cognitive function and more daytime sleepiness in chronic fatigue syndrome. Some side effects from medication or treatment may also induce sleepiness or an increase in fatigue, making naps necessary.

To summarise – as with everything else, it's about balance. If you are struggling to get enough hours' sleep at night, have a strict sleep-hygiene schedule and want to include the option of a nap during the day and that works for you, then naps aren't bad. If you are including a nap, I'd suggest taking it in the early afternoon, so it's not too close to the morning, but also not too close to bedtime (try not to nap past 4pm). Set a timer or alarm to wake you up, with your maximum nap time being between forty-five and ninety minutes. And once you wake up, try to sit in sunlight/daylight if possible, and do something active, so your body knows it is still daytime.

12

Exercising with pain

This chapter is for those of us who live alongside daily pain as part of our baseline functioning. Many of us living with autoimmune conditions are encouraged by others to wait to exercise until we feel better, or until a new treatment starts or until after certain tests. But the truth is, if we waited until our pain eased or until conditions were perfect before exercising, we would likely never do any.

It can be a challenge to differentiate between pain that means we are still in a safe zone and pain that means it is unsafe to exercise. How do we 'listen' to our bodies, while not obsessing about our pain? Finding a balance between ignoring versus listening to pain signals can feel impossible.

Understanding pain physiology – specifically chronic-pain physiology – really helps here. Recognising the function of pain can help us to identify what we need to pay attention to. Then we can use this to help us know when to exercise or rest, and sometimes even use exercise as a tool in managing pain.

Pain and the brain

When I was growing up, if any healthcare professional told me 'the pain is in your head', they were immediately crossed off my Christmas-card list. I found this approach dismissive of the extreme pain I was experiencing, and having spent years undiagnosed and, many times, not believed, any mention that I could be the one causing my pain and/or that I was making it up put me on the defensive. Couldn't they understand that there were things physically wrong with my body and causing pain? Didn't they realise I would do anything to live with less pain?

Now, many years on, and having studied pain physiology at university as part of my physiotherapy degree, as well as undertaking further courses in understanding pain and the nervous system, I do agree that pain 100 per cent comes from the brain – *but* it is also 100 per cent not your fault and the pain is still completely valid and real.

The brain, which is part of the central nervous system, constantly receives information from receptors throughout the body via neural pathways and sends messages back to tell each body part what to do. Its number-one priority is to keep us safe, and if it perceives something to be dangerous, it will send pain signals to notify us. So the pain response is from the brain's perception of what is happening and how much of a threat that could be. It acts like an alarm system, alerting us to actual or potential tissue damage. For example, if you misjudge chopping a carrot, and instead chop your finger, your brain will definitely tell you your finger was cut by the knife by screaming 'PAIN'. But equally, if you misjudged the carrot and only struck the chopping board, your brain might still perceive that you chopped your finger, and still send pain signals, despite there being no actual damage. In another scenario, if you did chop your finger because you were distracted by the fact that your whole kitchen was on fire, you wouldn't the feel finger pain, as at that moment your brain would be more threatened by the fire and focused on getting you safely out of there. The brain is constantly assessing everything to try to keep you safe.

According to David S. Butler and G. Lorimer Moseley in their book *Explain Pain*, 'The amount of pain you experience does not necessarily relate to the amount of tissue damage you have sustained'. Someone with back pain might have a scan showing a slipped disc or degenerative changes, but someone else without back pain could have a scan showing the same thing. Our pain relies heavily on context when interpreting sensory cues from around the body, including stress, emotions, knowledge, fears and beliefs around pain. Age, culture and gender also affect pain thresholds, which explains why pain is individual to each person. It cannot be compared or judged, as no two people have the exact same experience. For example, when I first had pain when I was younger, I was afraid of it. I had no diagnosis, and my pain was a constant alarm, telling me something was not right. I was fearful of doing the wrong thing and making it worse and, as a result, I became weaker and weaker, as I lost muscle strength. Once I understood my body and pain, however, the pain itself was less scary and I felt more in control of how I could help my body. Later, when I hurt my back, my perceptions of this pain were impacted by my previous experiences – I was scared of going back to being unable to walk again. I hadn't paid attention to the earlier whispers that my body was struggling, so the pain ramped up, until I had no choice but to stop and listen. I was unable to work, yet I needed to – and the pressure I put on myself and the stress regarding my situation amplified my pain further still. My brain perceived the loss of income, my visa and my flat as part of the pain picture associated with my back injury.

Acute pain is often easier to make sense of – such as in the carrot-chopping example above. The brain responds to a clear one-off event and sends pain signals as a result. Then, once the initial threat has receded, the tissues heal, the pain eases and you can carry on as normal. When the pain becomes chronic, however, it can feel harder to understand, making our relationship with our bodies and pain more complex. The underlying physiology remains the same, though: the brain has concluded that it feels under threat, and we must try to work out why and help it to feel safe again.

Pain becomes chronic when it lasts for longer than three months. At this stage, as the pain continues, the nervous system is highly attuned to danger alarms. Often called 'central sensitisation', the whole pain pathway becomes overactive and needs less and less input from the messenger neurons in the tissue in the first place in order to produce pain. All the systems in our bodies then start to become more involved and perpetuate the pain cycle. Our sympathetic nervous system, along with our adrenal glands, produce more adrenaline, and the endocrine system produces more cortisol (often known as a stress chemical), making our bodies feel stuck in 'fight or flight'. The immune system communicates with the sympathetic nervous system and endocrine system, which then releases pro-inflammatory chemicals called cytokines, which help to spread pain around other areas of the body or flare up old injuries. To summarise: every system in the body ramps up, responding as though everything is a constant threat and, as a result, the brain becomes very good at labelling everything as pain.

Movement and pain

Sometimes when the brain is trying to keep us safe, it can prime our muscles as part of our fight-or-flight response. This was useful in the prehistoric era, when we needed our bodies to be ready to sprint away from a sabre-toothed tiger. It's less helpful, though, when we have pain from an autoimmune flare. Chronic pain means we end up overusing certain bigger global muscles designed to help us run away from that tiger, but they tend to dominate and prevent us from using our smaller stabilising muscles as effectively. Sometimes the brain also has an inhibitory effect on our soft tissue, trying to 'freeze' to avoid further damage. This, again, leads to some muscles not being able to do their jobs as they were designed to.

One of the consequences of pain are changes in movement patterns. Perhaps your gait pattern is altered if you start to limp due to injury in one of your joints or you stop bending or moving in a certain way if you experience pain in your back. Over time, your options for movement become fewer, as your body has learned these new, less efficient motor patterns due to the pain. Then, because of how your body has adapted, this, in turn, can perpetuate the pain cycle, as soft tissues and joints are only being used in a certain way and the body does not like feeling stuck.

Movement can help with the effects of pain in several ways. It can actually help your brain to feel safe again. You can reteach it through changing the neural pathways to show that movement is good and beneficial for your body, rather than something to fear, to avoid or that will make your pain worse. So the idea is to reintegrate movement gradually (not too quickly, as that will create the same boom-and-bust pattern we talked about in the previous chapter), using exercise to manage pain, release any muscle imbalances and strengthen and support the body.

How do I know which pain is 'ok' and which is 'bad'?

As we now know, pain is not always an accurate measure of what is going on inside our bodies, but it should still be noticed and listened to. When you experience high or new pain, it's useful to check in with yourself and assess what this is telling you. Is it something new? Is it something that makes sense – for example, ankle pain after rolling your ankle? Does it correlate with how the rest of you feels – for example, autoimmune flare with joint pain, fevers and rashes? This kind of analytical thinking will help you to wade through the pain signals your brain is giving you and note when you need to seek help or when you can continue trying to manage the pain yourself.

In terms of exercising with pain, you need to respect it and find a way of working with it. If you try to beat it, ignore it and keep pushing, you'll flood your nervous system with danger chemicals and wipe yourself out – often for days, due to an increase in symptoms. Equally, if you try to avoid pain, stopping the moment you feel it start or ramp up, you'll end up being able to do less and less. The threshold of activity at which you feel pain reduces, and you are able to do less with the same or sometimes even more pain.

Hopefully, having now gained a clearer understanding of what pain is and, using the pain scenarios below, you will be better placed to assess and think through the strategies that are open to you. But of course, as always, it really does depend on your individual circumstances.

Baseline pain

This is your 'normal' pain. For some, their baseline level of pain may be no pain (I'm not jealous at all!), for others, it may be localised to a few specific areas and for others still, it could be widespread. In general, your baseline pain should allow you to carry out your usual activities of daily living, even if your level of function is reduced because of your pain and/or other factors like fatigue. Your exercise plan should be based on this level of pain.

Example: I have my usual pain, nothing is particularly 'loud' and I know that exercising is going to make me feel better and probably help with some of the pain.

New, unexplained pain

If it is something new that you have not experienced before, it is advised to have this assessed by someone from your healthcare team before continuing with exercise. This is not to automatically say that carrying on with exercise is wrong or unsafe, just that it is best practice to ensure you're not ignoring a red flag (such as a serious medical issue) – especially if the pain is severe, impacting your ability to carry out your usual activities of daily living and is not responding to methods that you would typically use to manage it. Depending on the severity of the unexplained pain and how this is impacting you, your healthcare team might decide to reduce your exercise plan or adapt it to work with your new pain.

Example: I have a sudden, right-sided, sharp pain in my stomach. It feels very different from the usual stomach pain I experience. Nothing I do is helping it and it feels like it is getting worse. I would try to see my doctor and focus on breathwork and trying to help the rest of my body relax as best as possible.

New, explained pain

In this scenario, you can explain the new pain – perhaps you stubbed your toe and now it hurts. You may choose to speak to someone in your medical team for support or advice on how to manage whatever is going on, especially if it is impacting your activities or is not controlled. And depending on the severity, and the explanation for the pain, it is likely that you'll need to adapt your usual plan to accommodate the problem for a short period.

Example: my knees have become red, hot and swollen (a typical sign of a lupus flare for me, especially with triggers like weather changes). I may decide to pull back my exercise plan to focus on moving my hip, knee and ankle joints, but in a low-impact way, and look at my total energy expenditure (activity cup – see pp. 56–9) to see if I can tweak it to help with the flare. If it continues, I may reach out to my medical team.

Higher-than-normal pain

This is when your pain is in the usual places and of the usual type, but higher than normal. Maybe it is impacting your daily activities more and you have already had to adapt your day's plan. You want to do your best to look at why your pain is higher and then adapt your exercise plan accordingly.

Example: I wake up with pain in the usual places, but it feels much higher than on an average day. I check in with myself to see what else could be contributing to this – such as, how much sleep I have had, how busy I have been, stress levels, any changes in medication or anything new I have added to my day-to-day routine. Depending on my findings, I may have a rest day or focus on breathwork, gentle mobility to support my body and see if I can help it feel more comfortable.

ADAPTING MOVEMENT FOR HIGHER-PAIN DAYS

You can see from my examples that having higher pain than normal does not always mean an automatic no to movement. As we've seen, movement can be helpful in managing pain or even easing it sometimes. That's not to say that you cannot rest – you totally can and with zero guilt – but there are ways to adapt exercise in response to higher-pain days should you want to. Here are some examples:

- Factoring in an extra rest day
- Doing fewer repetitions or sets
- Reducing the weight, load, resistance
- Changing the activity to something lighter
- Changing the position of how you exercise – for example, choosing lying over standing
- Factoring in more rest time before, during and after the activity
- Reducing other physical activity during the day to prioritise exercise
- Focusing on gentle mobility movements or breathwork

Usual pain worsens *with* exercise

If your usual pain worsens when you start to move, you should pause and assess what's going on. Return to a position that feels comfortable while you check in with yourself. Try not to catastrophise, as this will create a negative spiral, amplifying the pain signals. Instead, bring yourself to a state of calm, observing the sensations in your body. Perhaps use whatever pain-management techniques you find helpful (see p. 225) or keep it simple and focus on your breath. Once you feel ready, see if you can repeat the movement, perhaps moving more slowly or through a smaller range. Notice how this feels. If the pain continues, try another exercise and see how that feels. If your brain is labelling everything as pain today, maybe you're just not in a physical or mental state to exercise in this moment. Perhaps you have missed something your body is trying to communicate and you need to support it in other ways first (such as through rest), rather than through movement.

If you suffer with migraine attacks, you may find that movement sometimes aggravates your pain, in which case stop. It may not be what your body needs in that moment. Everyone responds differently to migraine – for me, movement with an attack exacerbates my pain and nausea. But I usually find at the end of an attack that I can tolerate some gentle mobility exercises to help me reconnect to myself as I recover.

Usual pain is worse *after* exercising

If your pain is much worse *after* exercising and takes a while to come back down again or impacts your ability to do other activities, it probably means your exercise plan needs to be changed. Feeling muscle soreness afterwards is common, but high pain that impacts your function is not what you are after. You are trying to tell the brain it is safe to move and encourage production of the chemicals that reduce the pain response. Too much too soon can trigger a higher pain response and an increase in inflammation. It takes time to build up slowly and increase resilience and tolerance to movement. You need to pick the dosage of movement that is right for your body in that moment.

Flare-up from exercise

If you do flare up by doing 'too much' or something your body was unable cope with, the most important thing is not to panic. I know that's easier said than done. An injury or increase in pain can remind you of past experiences – the uncertainty, the trauma and the journey you have been on to get you where you are today. It's easy to jump straight back there mentally and panic that you will lose all the progress you've made and be back at square one. But panicking will just make your pain worse – your brain will think, Oh my gosh! I am right – something is *really* wrong. And it will increase those pain signals. Remember, your nervous system is on high alert and is very sensitive, so it does not take much to tip it over the edge from, 'I've got this' to, 'Aahhh – I haven't got this'. Do not give yourself a hard time or feel guilty. It is not your fault. You are human, and walking this fine line of doing enough but not too much with chronic illness is tricky. Your brain is trying its best to protect you, so be compassionate towards yourself, use your toolbox (see p. 225) to help you manage this temporary flare and then build back up again, slowly and consistently.

How to help your pain

Understanding pain is key, as is trying to support the body's systems to calm down and feel safe. The autonomic nervous system (ANS) balances its two branches, the sympathetic nervous system (SNS, aka fight or flight) and parasympathetic nervous system (PNS, aka rest and digest), to help our bodies react in an appropriate way – for example, increasing heart rate for exercise or calming the body to help it sleep. Pain makes the SNS louder and more in control, so we want to support the PNS to be more active, too, creating that sense of calm and relaxation to tell the brain it is safe. Tools that help with this are sometimes described as 'safety in me' or 'glimmers', compared to activities that ramp up pain or the SNS, which can be called 'danger in me' or 'triggers'. The idea is to build up a toolbox of 'safety in me' and 'glimmers' to help manage pain by activating the PNS.

OUR NERVOUS SYSTEM

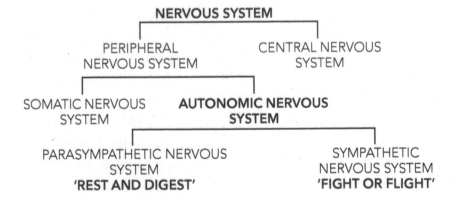

On high pain days, it can be really hard to remember anything useful, as all the brain can think about is safety. It can be helpful at those times to have a list to remind you of supportive tools that are in your control to help.

Building your toolbox is personal, as different approaches or tools work for different people, so it's about playing around with options. I find different tools are needed for different types of pain, too. For example, breathwork is so helpful for bladder pain, but I find it is much harder to reach for during a migraine attack.

Your pain-management toolbox

Here are some ideas to keep in mind whenever you need some extra support with pain:

- Gentle exercise
- Breathwork
- Ice or heat, warm baths
- Neuromodulation devices (like TENS machines)
- Rest
- Acupressure mat
- Calm activities you enjoy – for example, being creative, doing a puzzle, cuddling a pet
- Aromatherapy
- Meditation, tapping or mindfulness
- Gentle massage devices

VAGUS NERVE

The vagus nerve is our tenth cranial nerve and acts like a busy motorway, carrying information to and from the body's systems. It is the main component of the para-sympathetic system which helps the body to be in the 'rest-and-digest' state. Vagus-nerve activity has been shown to inhibit inflammation, reduce oxidative stress and calm the sympathetic nervous system (fight or flight). It is thought to have a role in helping with pain, and a number of studies have looked at vagus-nerve-stimulation devices as pain-management tools. You can also stimulate your vagus nerve with deep breathing, laughter, cold-water exposure, exercise or even singing!

Exercising with pain

Understanding your pain and nervous system will help you to work with them – listening to your body without feeling overwhelmed by pain and helping you to feel more empowered to manage it through movement and other pain management tools.

13

Mindset and movement

Our mindsets around movement can be one of the biggest challenges to overcome.

Our relationship with exercise starts in childhood – our exposure to discussion around it, our role models and the options we had available to us. These experiences shape our beliefs of how we value and/or appreciate movement.

For some, exercise has never been easy. Maybe you were the last in races or found sport challenging. Perhaps you didn't enjoy it and maybe you built a mental block, telling yourself, 'I can't do this' or, 'I am rubbish at exercising'. A lot of our enjoyment can come from being good at something, so if you never found something you were naturally skilled at or could practise enough to build your skill level, this could be why. It also may relate to health issues – maybe you have always struggled with your fitness, which, on reflection, is why you found running so hard. My mum never realised she was hypermobile until my diagnosis, and for her this was so validating, following her difficult experiences with sport at school. Sometimes we can look back and join the dots to understand why our bodies have always struggled with certain things.

On the other end of the spectrum, I loved exercise. I was used to pushing myself with training and challenging myself at competitions. Losing that part of myself when I was first unable to exercise came with a huge amount of grief. Then came several boom-and-bust years, when I sought that same gratification from pushing myself. Over time, I learned how to adapt exercise to work with my body and my conditions – and with that, I had to change my mindset, too. That all-or-nothing mindset of what 'counts' as exercise had to be undone. I had to learn patience with setbacks, again and again. I had to learn compassion for myself – because even when I felt I had lowered my expectations of what exercise could be, my body could still not manage that. I had to try to stop comparing myself to those around me, whether healthy and abled or others with my conditions. Most importantly, I had to stop making comparisons with my past self. I had to process the grief for what I was able to do previously and feel gratitude for what I am able to do now.

Society, TV shows, the press and social media do not help with supporting a healthy mindset around activity. It can be so difficult to search and choose between the millions of options out there, filtering the fact from the pseudoscience. Exercise can often be incorrectly labelled as 'low impact' or 'easy' or 'beginner level' when it includes advanced or high-impact exercises. That then creates a narrative in which people tell themselves they're not good enough, feeling weak and rubbish about themselves, when really, the activity they were doing was just not the right level for them.

All too often, exercise is aimed at pushing you to the point where you need to be red, sweaty and trembling with DOMS (see p. 187) for days. In fact, it has been proven that these are not useful indicators of how hard you have worked. Even healthy individuals get burnt out with high-intensity workouts and trying to achieve arbitrary goals, regardless of how they feel.

So here, we are trying to change your narrative of how movement looks, feels and is for you. Sometimes you have to dig deep and do the work to help process past trauma or challenge past beliefs. Sometimes that can mean unfollowing certain social media accounts or leaving a gym because of the unhelpful language or beliefs they share. Sometimes it's just a matter of tuning into your self-talk and noticing how you speak to yourself about movement and your body. A lot of my clients are highly critical of their own bodies. How many of the following (or similar) do you find yourself saying?

- My body is broken
- I have a bad knee
- I have rubbish posture
- I have lazy glutes
- I have a weird walk
- My muscles are useless
- My body is a failure

Don't get me wrong; I am not implying you have to be positive all the time about your body. You are absolutely allowed to say when life sucks. This is just about trying to bring awareness to how you are describing your body and the language you use, often without realising.

Firstly, it's rarely one body part that is at fault. Calling your knee 'bad' is like blaming one child for talking when the whole class was talking, too. Plus, your glutes (nor any other muscle) would never just decide to be lazy for no reason. Our bodies are incredibly clever and complex. It requires multiple organs and systems to co-ordinate in a millisecond, just for us to be able to move a single body part. So there is always a reason why your body behaves the way it does. It could be a protective mechanism at play, like we discussed in the pain chapter, or maybe it's an adaptation from an injury years ago. Whatever it is, your body is trying its absolute best 24/7 to keep you safe.

When we are in pain, and the brain is very worried about a potential or an actual threat, it can make us more critical of ourselves. Then, constantly referring to body parts using negative terminology can perpetuate the messaging that something is wrong. Usually, wrong = more pain. And so the cycle continues.

Of course, this isn't to say that if you talk about your back injury using terms of endearment, it will magically heal. (That would be great, but we know pain is more complex than this.) But research has found self-compassion to be a useful therapy in chronic pain, showing benefits in how we cope and, as a result improve, our mental wellbeing.

I went on a self-compassion journey a couple of years after my lupus diagnosis and found it incredibly helpful to change my thought pathways through the way I spoke to myself. I would be mean about being mean to myself: 'Are you stupid? Why can't you be more self-compassionate?' This helped me across all areas in life, but particularly around acceptance of my health and with exercise. If I wasn't well enough to move my body, I would no longer beat myself up about it. I would respect my body for telling me and be kind to myself. I stopped fighting rest as well. I used to say I was lazy, unproductive or weak for needing a rest, whereas now, my afternoon rest has become a game changer in my ability to function.

Acceptance is weird with any chronic condition. I think it is less of an endpoint and more of a work in progress. Just when you think you have successfully navigated accepting your baseline, something changes and suddenly, you are faced with thoughts you did not think you'd have to deal with. There are layers, and as you peel away one, facing you is another to slowly work through. Pain psychology enabled me to understand my body and what it is trying to tell me. Therapy was a neutral space in which to process some of the medical trauma I had collected over the years and give me strategies to support my mental health, in the same way I have my toolbox to support my physical health. Time has helped me to grow wiser and, with that, to accept my reality with compassion and understanding. To expect yourself to be able to tick off 'accept chronic illness' or 'be kind to myself' from your to-do list in a day is unrealistic. It takes time, but this is the start of your journey of relearning and accepting how to move in a way that works for you.

MOVEMENT AND MINDSET FRAMEWORK

1. How do you currently feel about exercise (for example, frustrated)?
2. How do you want to feel about exercise (for example, positive, relaxed, in control)?
3. What beliefs or feelings are preventing you from feeling that way (if, for example, you still compare yourself to your past self and what you were able to do).
4. How can you support yourself to feel the way you want to around movement (for example, focusing on what you can do in this moment, being self-compassionate, rather than negative towards yourself over what you cannot do)?
5. What do you think your biggest mindset barriers are to movement, and can you think of an action plan for overcoming each one? (Perhaps you feel like you can't do much, so you tell yourself, there is no point.) Action plan: remind yourself of your 'why' – see p. 29 – and that all movement counts; set yourself a small target, say, one exercise, and remind yourself that that is enough.

Final words

I hope you have taken away lots of practical advice on how to *actually* exercise with an autoimmune condition. Some of the changes you make might be big or bold, while others might be small tweaks to your routine. It will take time for the exercises you add in to build awareness in your body, improve your stability and strengthen your muscles. But overall, this is going to improve your everyday ability to function.

Living with a long-term health condition can reduce the options available to you, making your world smaller, whether that is with everyday tasks, socially, with work or for fun. Through movement, however, you can open those options up again and, as a result, expand your world. Movement helps to create a feeling of connection and safety back in your body and after experiencing pain and medical trauma, you really need your body to feel like a safe home again.

So many clients come to me already feeling like they have failed to exercise with their condition and blaming themselves. It's hard to be consistent with exercise for anyone. But perhaps more so when living with a fluctuating condition – from when you first experience symptoms and feel lost among tests and appointments, to trying to understand what is happening in your body. From when you are first diagnosed and are, perhaps, unsure of what your future may look like, to starting some form of treatment (maybe several) and coping with the yo-yo of side effects and withdrawals. To then changing your mindset and views on what exercise 'used' to look like, letting go of beliefs about what it 'should' be like and comparing what you can do to what others can manage. It might sound clichéd, but this truly is a journey – to find a balance and understand how best to exercise for you and your body.

So take some pressure off. Be kind to yourself and regularly remind yourself you are enough, wherever you are on this road. My mantra here is 'Do what you can, when you can' – and I think this really sums up how to exercise with autoimmunity. Perhaps I didn't need to write a whole book, after all!

Resources

Pain

Explain Pain by David Butler and Lorimer Moseley (Adelaide: Noigroup Publications, 2013)

The Pain Management Workbook by Dr Rachel Zoffness (Oakland, CA: New Harbinger Publications, 2020)

The Brain That Changes Itself by Norman Doidge (London: Penguin, 2008)

The Way Out by Alan Gordon (London: Ebury, 2021)

Atomic Habits by James Clear (London: Cornerstone, 2018)

Retrain Pain website: www.retrainpain.org – a free resource on understanding pain

Curable app – includes education about chronic pain, cognitive behavioural therapy techniques and meditations to help manage pain

Headspace app – meditation and mindfulness tools, with some courses specifically on sleep and pain

Calm app – meditation and mindfulness, with guided and unguided sessions

Balance app – meditation, with tailored programmes, depending on your skill and experience

The Tapping Solution app – tapping, or emotional freedom technique, is a form of acupressure to help with calming the nervous system

Online exercise for autoimmune conditions

Yoga for AS – www.yogaforas.com – yoga modified for ankylosing spondylitis

Yoga Dr Nikki – www.yogadrnikki.com – Dr Nikki is a rheumatologist and yoga instructor specialising in tailoring yoga for those with autoimmune conditions

The MSing Link – www.doctorgretchenhawley.com – Dr Gretchen Hawley is a physiotherapist specialising in helping those with multiple sclerosis to exercise and feel more confident in their strength, walking and daily activities

Online tai chi – www.taichionlineclasses.com – Dr Paul Lam has a series of online videos ranging from beginner sessions to specific conditions like diabetes and arthritis

YouTube – there are lots of great free resources here on exercising with chronic pain and autoimmune conditions

Condition-specific associations or charities (for example, Lupus UK, Versus Arthritis, MS Society, Crohn's and Colitis Foundation to name a few) often have great resources and free video libraries of starter exercises

PAR-Q - www.eparmedx.com

References

Introduction

- Bierman, A. S., Wang, J., O'Malley, P. G. & Moss, D. K. (2021). 'Transforming care for people with multiple chronic conditions: Agency for Healthcare Research and Quality's research agenda.' *Health Services Research*, 56 (Suppl 1), 973–9. https://doi.org/10.1111/1475-6773.13863
- Kadakia, S., Stratton, C., Wu, Y., Feliciano, J. & Tuakli-Wosornu, Y. A. (2022). 'The Accessibility of YouTube Fitness Videos for Individuals Who Are Disabled Before and During the COVID-19 Pandemic: Preliminary Application of a Text Analytics Approach.' *JMIR Formative Research*, 6(2), e34176. https://doi.org/10.2196/34176
- Jacqueline, I. (2018). *Surviving and Thriving with an Invisible Chronic Illness: How to Stay Sane and Live One Step Ahead of Your Symptoms*. New Harbinger Publications.
- Hunt, E. R. & Papathomas, A. (2020). 'Being physically active through chronic illness: Life experiences of people with arthritis.' *Qualitative Research in Sport, Exercise and Health*, 12(2), 242–55. https://doi.org/10.1080/2159676X.2019.1601637

Chapter 2: The benefits of exercising with autoimmune conditions

- Bull, F. C., Al-Ansari, S. S., Biddle, S., Borodulin, K., Buman, M. P., Cardon, G., Carty, C., Chaput, J. P., Chastin, S., Chou, R., Dempsey, P. C., DiPietro, L., Ekelund, U., Firth, J., Friedenreich, C. M., Garcia, L., Gichu, M., Jago, R., Katzmarzyk, P. T., Lambert, E., . . . Willumsen, J. F. (2020). 'World Health Organization 2020 guidelines on physical activity and sedentary behaviour.' *British Journal of Sports Medicine*, 54(24), 1451–62. https://doi.org/10.1136/bjsports-2020-102955
- 'WHO guidelines on physical activity and sedentary behaviour: Web Annex. Evidence profiles.' Geneva: World Health Organization; 2020. Licence: CC BY-NC-SA 3.0 IGO. Available at: https://apps.who.int/iris/bitstream/handle/10665/336657/9789240015111-eng.pdf?utm_medium=email&utm_source=transaction
- Brukner, P. D. & Brown, W. J. (2005). '3. Is exercise good for you?' *Medical Journal of Australia*, 183(10), 538–41. https://doi.org/10.5694/j.1326-5377.2005.tb07159.x
- Gualano, B., Pinto, A. L., Perondi, M. B., Roschel, H., Sallum, A. M., Hayashi, A. P., Solis, M. Y. & Silva, C. A. (2011). 'Therapeutic effects of exercise training in patients with pediatric rheumatic diseases.' *Revista brasileira de reumatologia*, 51(5), 490–6. https://www.scielo.br/j/rbr/a/W7Myq3Z7vKwBDgSYjCdc9Rm/?lang=en#ModalTutors
- Metsios, G. S., Moe, R. H., & Kitas, G. D. (2020). 'Exercise and inflammation.' *Best Practice & Research: Clinical Rheumatology*, 34(2), 101504. https://doi.org/10.1016/j.berh.2020.101504

- Sharif, K., Watad, A., Bragazzi, N. L., Lichtbroun, M., Amital, H., & Shoenfeld, Y. (2018). 'Physical activity and autoimmune diseases: Get moving and manage the disease.' *Autoimmunity Reviews*, 17(1), 53–72. https://doi.org/10.1016/j. autrev.2017.11.010

- Xie, Y. & Wang, J. P. (2019). 'Sheng li xue bao': [Acta physiologica Sinica], 71(5), 769–82. Available at: https://pubmed. ncbi.nlm.nih.gov/31646331/

- Metsios, G. S. & Kitas, G. D. (2018). 'Physical activity, exercise and rheumatoid arthritis: Effectiveness, mechanisms and implementation.' *Best Practice & Research: Clinical Rheumatology*, 32(5), 669–82. https://doi. org/10.1016/j.berh.2019.03.013

- Mendes Sieczkowska, S., Infante Smaira, F., Caruso Mazzolani, B., Gualano, B., Roschel, H. & Peçanha, T. (2021). 'Efficacy of home-based physical activity interventions in patients with autoimmune rheumatic diseases: A systematic review and meta-analysis.' *Seminars in Arthritis and Rheumatism*, 51(3), 576–87. ISSN 0049-0172. https://doi.org/10.1016/j.semarthrit.2021.04.004

- Perandini, L. A., de Sá-Pinto, A. L., Roschel, H., Benatti, F. B., Lima, F. R., Bonfá, E. & Gualano, B. (2012). 'Exercise as a therapeutic tool to counteract inflammation and clinical symptoms in autoimmune rheumatic diseases.' *Autoimmunity Reviews*, 12(2), 218–24. https://doi.org/10.1016/j. autrev.2012.06.007

- Thomas J. L. (2013). 'Helpful or harmful? Potential effects of exercise on select inflammatory conditions.' *The Physician and Sportsmedicine*, 41(4), 93–100. https://doi.org/10.3810/ psm.2013.11.2040

References

- Gualano, B., Sá Pinto, A. L., Perondi, B., Leite Prado, D. M., Omori, C., Almeida, R. T., Sallum, A. M. & Silva, C. A. (2010). 'Evidence for prescribing exercise as treatment in pediatric rheumatic diseases.' *Autoimmunity Reviews*, 9(8), 569–73. https://doi.org/10.1016/j.autrev.2010.04.001

- Cooney, J. K., Law, R. J., Matschke, V., Lemmey, A. B., Moore, J. P., Ahmad, Y., Jones, J. G., Maddison, P. & Thom, J. M. (2011). 'Benefits of exercise in rheumatoid arthritis.' *Journal of Aging Research*, 2011, 681640. https://doi.org/10.4061/2011/681640

- Ottawa Panel (2004). 'Ottawa Panel evidence-based clinical practice guidelines for therapeutic exercises in the management of rheumatoid arthritis in adults.' *Physical Therapy*, 84(10), 934–72. Available at: https://pubmed.ncbi.nlm.nih.gov/15449978/

- De Jong, Z., Munneke, M., Zwinderman, A. H., Kroon, H. M., Jansen, A., Ronday, K. H., van Schaardenburg, D., Dijkmans, B. A., Van den Ende, C. H., Breedveld, F. C., Vliet Vlieland, T. P. & Hazes, J. M. (2003). 'Is a long-term high-intensity exercise program effective and safe in patients with rheumatoid arthritis? Results of a randomized controlled trial.' *Arthritis and Rheumatology*, 48(9), 2415–24. https://doi.org/10.1002/art.11216

- Rodrigues, R., Ferraz, R. B., Kurimori, C. O., Guedes, L. K., Lima, F. R., de Sá-Pinto, A. L., Gualano, B. & Roschel, H. (2019). 'Low-Load Resistance Training With Blood-Flow Restriction in Relation to Muscle Function, Mass, and Functionality in Women With Rheumatoid Arthritis.' *Arthritis Care & Research*, 71(5), 679–87. https://doi.org/10.1002/acr.23911

- Halabchi, F., Alizadeh, Z., Sahraian, M. A. & Abolhasani, M. (2017). 'Exercise prescription for patients with multiple sclerosis; potential benefits and practical recommendations.' *BMC Neurology*, 17(1), 185. https://doi.org/10.1186/s12883-017-0960-9

- Pilutti, L. A., Platta, M. E., Motl, R. W. & Latimer-Cheung, A. E. (2014). 'The safety of exercise training in multiple sclerosis: a systematic review.' *Journal of the Neurological Sciences*, 343(1–2), 3–7. https://doi.org/10.1016/j.jns.2014.05.016
- Motl, R. W. & Sandroff, B. M. (2015). 'Benefits of Exercise Training in Multiple Sclerosis.' *Current Neurology and Neuroscience Reports*, 15(9), 62. https://doi.org/10.1007/s11910-015-0585-6
- White, L. J., McCoy, S. C., Castellano, V., Gutierrez, G., Stevens, J. E., Walter, G. A. & Vandenborne, K. (2004). 'Resistance training improves strength and functional capacity in persons with multiple sclerosis.' *Multiple Sclerosis Journal*, 10(6), 668–74. https://doi.org/10.1191/1352458504ms1088oa
- Ayán, C. & Martín, V. (2007). 'Systemic lupus erythematosus and exercise.' *Lupus*, 16(1), 5–9. https://doi.org/10.1177/0961203306074795
- Ayán, C., de Pedro-Múñez, A., & Martínez-Lemos, I. (2018). 'Efectos del ejercicio físico en personas con lupus eritematoso sistémico: revisión sistemática' ['Effects of physical exercise in a population with systemic lupus erythematosus: A systematic review']. *Semergen*, 44(3), 192–206. https://doi.org/10.1016/j.semerg.2017.12.002
- Keramiotou, K., Anagnostou, C., Kataxaki, E., et al. (2020). 'The impact of upper limb exercise on function, daily activities, and quality of life in systemic lupus erythematosus: A pilot randomized controlled trial.' *RMD Open*, 6, e001141. https://doi.org/10.1136/rmdopen-2019-001141

References

- Tench, C., Bentley, D., Vleck, V., McCurdie, I., White, P. & D'Cruz, D. (2002). 'Aerobic fitness, fatigue, and physical disability in systemic lupus erythematosus.' *Journal of Rheumatology*, 29(3), 474–81. https://pubmed.ncbi.nlm.nih.gov/11908559/

- Balsamo, S. & Santos-Neto, L. D. (2011). 'Fatigue in systemic lupus erythematosus: An association with reduced physical fitness.' *Autoimmunity Reviews*, 10(9), 514–18. https://doi.org/10.1016/j.autrev.2011.03.005

- Maidhof, W. & Hilas, O. (2012). 'Lupus: An overview of the disease and management options.' *Pharmacy and Therapeutics*, 37(4), 240–49. Available at: https://www.ncbi.nlm.nih.gov/pmc/articles/PMC3351863/

- Ayán, C. & Martín, V. (2007). 'Systemic lupus erythematosus and exercise.' *Lupus*, 16(1), 5–9. https://doi.org/10.1177/0961203306074795

- Tench, C., Bentley, D., Vleck, V., McCurdie, I., White, P. & D'Cruz, D. (2002). 'Aerobic fitness, fatigue, and physical disability in systemic lupus erythematosus.' *Journal of Rheumatology*, 29(3), 474–81. Available at: https://pubmed.ncbi.nlm.nih.gov/11908559/

- Perandini, L. A., V. Mello, S. B., Camara, N. O., Benatti, F. B., Lima, F. R., Borba, E., Bonfa, E., Sá-Pinto, A. L., Roschel, H. & Gualano, B. (2014). 'Exercise training can attenuate the inflammatory milieu in women with systemic lupus erythematosus.' *Journal of Applied Physiology*, 117(6), 639–47. https://doi.org/10.1152/japplphysiol.00486.2014

- Warburton, D. E., Nicol, C. W.' & Bredin, S. S. (2006). 'Health benefits of physical activity: the evidence.' *Canadian Medical Association Journal*, 174(6), 801–9. https://doi.org/10.1503/cmaj.051351

- Hasanpour Dehkordi A. (2016). 'Influence of yoga and aerobics exercise on fatigue, pain and psychosocial status in patients with multiple sclerosis: a randomized trial.' *Journal of Sports Medicine and Physical Fitness*, 56(11), 1417–22. Available at: https://pubmed.ncbi.nlm.nih.gov/26223004/

- Antunes, M. D. & Marques, A. P. (2022). 'The role of physiotherapy in fibromyalgia: Current and future perspectives.' *Frontiers in Physiology*, 13, 968292. https://doi.org/10.3389/fphys.2022.968292

- McDowell, C., Farooq, U. & Haseeb, M. (2023, April 16). 'Inflammatory Bowel Disease. In StatPearls [Internet]. Treasure Island, FL: StatPearls Publishing. Available at: https://www.ncbi.nlm.nih.gov/books/NBK470312/?report=reader#_NBK470312_pubdet_

- Grayston, R., Czanner, G., Elhadd, K., Goebel, A., Frank, B., Üçeyler, N., Malik, R. A. & Alam, U. (2019). 'A systematic review and meta-analysis of the prevalence of small fiber pathology in fibromyalgia: Implications for a new paradigm in fibromyalgia etiopathogenesis.' *Seminars in Arthritis and Rheumatism*, 48(5), 933–40. https://doi.org/10.1016/j.semarthrit.2018.08.003

- Goebel, A., Krock, E., Gentry, C., Israel, M. R., Jurczak, A., Urbina, C. M., Sandor, K., Vastani, N., Maurer, M., Cuhadar, U., Sensi, S., Nomura, Y., Menezes, J., Baharpoor, A., Brieskorn, L., Sandström, A., Tour, J., Kadetoff, D., Haglund, L., Kosek, E. . . . Andersson, D. A. (2021). 'Passive transfer of fibromyalgia symptoms from patients to mice.' *Journal of Clinical Investigation*, 131(13), e144201. https://doi.org/10.1172/JCI144201

- Busch, A. J., Webber, S. C., Brachaniec, M., Bidonde, J., Dal Bello-Haas, V., Danyliw, A. D., Overend, T. J., Richards, R.

S., Sawant, A. & Schachter, C. L. (2011). 'Exercise Therapy for Fibromyalgia.' *Current Pain and Headache Reports*, 15, 358–67. https://doi.org/10.1007/s11916-011-0214-2.

- Sosa-Reina, M. D., Nunez-Nagy, S., Gallego-Izquierdo, T., Pecos-Martín, D., Monserrat, J. & Álvarez-Mon, M. (2017). 'Effectiveness of Therapeutic Exercise in Fibromyalgia Syndrome: A Systematic Review and Meta-Analysis of Randomized Clinical Trials.' *BioMed Research International*, 2017, 2356346. https://doi.org/10.1155/2017/2356346

- Engels, M., Cross, R. K. & Long, M. D. (2017). 'Exercise in patients with inflammatory bowel diseases: current perspectives.' *Clinical and Experimental Gastroenterology*, 11, 1–11. https://doi.org/10.2147/CEG.S120816

- Holik, D., Včev, A., Milostić-Srb, A., Salinger, Ž., Ivanišević, Z., Včev, I., & Miškulin, M. (2019). 'The Effect of Daily Physical Activity on the Activity of Inflammatory Bowel Diseases in Therapy-Free Patients.' *Acta Clinica Croatica*, 58(2), 202–12. https://doi.org/10.20471/acc.2019.58.02.02

- Bilski, J., Brzozowski, B., Mazur-Bialy, A., Sliwowski, Z. & Brzozowski, T. (2014). 'The role of physical exercise in inflammatory bowel disease.' *BioMed Research International*, 2014, 429031. https://doi.org/10.1155/2014/429031

- Klasson, C. L., Sadhir, S. & Pontzer, H. (2022). 'Daily physical activity is negatively associated with thyroid hormone levels, inflammation, and immune system markers among men and women in the NHANES dataset.' *PLOS One*, 17(7), e0270221. https://doi.org/10.1371/journal.pone.0270221

- Ciloglu, F., Peker, I., Pehlivan, A., Karacabey, K., Ilhan, N., Saygin, O. & Ozmerdivenli, R. (2005). 'Exercise intensity and its effects on thyroid hormones.' *Neuroendocrinology*

Letters, 26(6), 830–4. Available at: https://pubmed.ncbi.nlm.nih.gov/16380698/

- Cutovic, M., Konstantinovic, L., Stankovic, Z. & Vesovic-Potic, V. (2012). 'Structured exercise program improves functional capacity and delays relapse in euthyroid patients with Graves' disease.' *Disability and Rehabilitation*, 34(18), 1511–18. https://doi.org/10.3109/09638288.2012.660599

- Werneck, F. Z., Coelho, E. F., Almas, S. P., Garcia, M. M. D. N., Bonfante, H. L. M., Lima, J. R. P., Vigário, P. D. S., Mainenti, M. R. M., Teixeira, P. F. D. S. & Vaisman, M. (2018). 'Exercise training improves quality of life in women with subclinical hypothyroidism: a randomized clinical trial.' *Archives of Endocrinology and Metabolism*, 62(5), 530–6. https://doi.org/10.20945/2359-3997000000073

- Bansal, A., Kaushik, A., Singh, C. M., Sharma, V. & Singh, H. (2015). 'The effect of regular physical exercise on the thyroid function of treated hypothyroid patients: An interventional study at a tertiary care center in Bastar region of India.' *Archives of Medicine and Health Sciences*, 3(2), 244–6. https://doi.org/10.4103/2321-4848.171913

- Galassetti, P. & Riddell, M. C. (2013). 'Exercise and type 1 diabetes (T1DM).' *Comprehensive Physiology*, 3(3), 1309–36. https://doi.org/10.1002/cphy.c110040

- Riddell, M. C., Gallen, I. W., Smart, C. E., Taplin, C. E., Adolfsson, P., Lumb, A. N., Kowalski, A., Rabasa-Lhoret, R., McCrimmon, R. J., Hume, C., Annan, F., Fournier, P. A., Graham, C., Bode, B., Galassetti, P., Jones, T. W., Millán, I. S., Heise, T., Peters, A. L., Petz, A. . . . Laffel, L. M. (2017). 'Exercise management in type 1 diabetes: a consensus statement.' *The Lancet. Diabetes & Endocrinology*, 5(5), 377–390. https://doi.org/10.1016/S2213-8587(17)30014-1

- Riddell, M. & Perkins, B. (2006). 'Type 1 Diabetes and Vigorous Exercise: Applications of Exercise Physiology to Patient Management.' *Canadian Journal of Diabetes*, 30. https://doi.org/10.1016/S1499-2671(06)01010-0.
- Riddell, M. C. & Iscoe, K. E. (2006). 'Physical activity, sport, and pediatric diabetes.' *Pediatric Diabetes*, 7(1), 60–70. https://doi.org/10.1111/j.1399-543X.2006.00146.x

Chapter 3: Goals and motivation

- Swann, C., Jackman, P. C., Lawrence, A., Hawkins, R. M., Goddard, S. G. & Williamson, O. (2022). 'The (over)use of SMART goals for physical activity promotion: A narrative review and critique.' *International Review of Sport and Exercise Psychology*, 15(2), 211–26. https://doi.org/10.1080/17437199.2021.2023608
- Hawkins, R. M., Crust, L., Swann, C. & Jackman, P. C. (2020). 'The effects of goal types on psychological outcomes in active and insufficiently active adults in a walking task: Further evidence for open goals.' *Psychology of Sport and Exercise*, 48, 101661. https://doi.org/10.1016/j.psychsport.2020.101661
- Anson, D. & Madras, D. (2016). 'Do low step count goals inhibit walking behavior: A randomized controlled study.' *Clinical Rehabilitation*, 30(7), 676–85. https://doi.org/10.1177/0269215515593782
- Clear, J. (2018). *Atomic Habits: An Easy & Proven Way to Build Good Habits & Break Bad Ones*. Avery.
- Duhigg, C. (2012). *The Power of Habit: Why We Do What We Do in Life and Business*. Random House.

- Neal, D. T., Wood, W., Labrecque, J. S. & Lally, P. (2012). 'How do habits guide behaviour? Perceived and actual triggers of habits in daily life.' *Journal of Experimental Social Psychology*, 48(2), 492–8. https://doi.org/10.1016/j.jesp.2011.10.011
- Lally, P., van Jaarsveld, C. H. M., Potts, H. W. W. & Wardle, J. (2009). 'How are habits formed: Modelling habit formation in the real world.' *European Journal of Social Psychology*, 40(6), 998–1009. https://doi.org/10.1002/ejsp.674
- Gardner, B., Lally, P. & Wardle, J. (2012). 'Making health habitual: the psychology of "habit-formation" and general practice.' *British Journal of General Practice*, 62(605), 664–6. https://doi.org/10.3399/bjgp12X659466
- Teixeira, P. J., Carraça, E. V., Markland, D., Silva, M. N. & Ryan, R. M. (2012). 'Exercise, physical activity, and self-determination theory: a systematic review.' *International Journal of Behavioral Nutrition and Physical Activity*, 9, 78. https://doi.org/10.1186/1479-5868-9-78

Chapter 5: Contraindications to exercise

- Astley, C., Pinto, A. J., Bonfá, E., da Silva, C. A. A. & Gualano, B. (2021). 'Gaps on rheumatologists' knowledge of physical activity.' *Clinical Rheumatology*, 40(7), 2907–11. https://doi.org/10.1007/s10067-020-05540-3
- Iversen, M. D., Fossel, A. H. & Daltroy, L. H. (1999). 'Rheumatologist-patient communication about exercise and physical therapy in the management of rheumatoid arthritis.' *Arthritis Care and Research : the official journal of the Arthritis Health Professions Association*, 12(3), 180–92. https://doi.org/10.1002/1529-0131(199906)12:3<180::aid-art5>3.0.co;2-#

References

- Gualano, B., Sá Pinto, A. L., Perondi, B., Prado, D. M. L., Omori, C., Almeida, R. T., Sallum, A. M. E. & Almeida Silva, C. A. (2010). 'Evidence for prescribing exercise as treatment in pediatric rheumatic diseases.' *Autoimmunity Reviews*, 9(8), 569–73. ISSN 1568-9972. https://doi.org/10.1016/j.autrev.2010.04.001

- Parry, S. M. & Puthucheary, Z. A. (2015). 'The impact of extended bed rest on the musculoskeletal system in the critical care environment.' *Extreme Physiology & Medicine*, 4, 16. https://doi.org/10.1186/s13728-015-0036-7

- Tazreean, R., Nelson, G. & Twomey, R. (2022). 'Early mobilization in enhanced recovery after surgery pathways: current evidence and recent advancements.' *Journal of Comparative Effectiveness Research*, 11(2), 121–9. https://doi.org/10.2217/cer-2021-0258

- Duncan, M. J., Rosenkranz, R. R., Vandelanotte, C., Caperchione, C. M., Rebar, A. L., Maeder, A. J., Tague, R., Savage, T. N., van Itallie, A., Mummery, W. K. & Kolt, G. S. (2016). 'What is the impact of obtaining medical clearance to participate in a randomized controlled trial examining a physical activity intervention on the socio-demographic and risk factor profiles of included participants?' *Trials*, 17, 580. https://doi.org/10.1186/s13063-016-1715-4

- Warburton, D. E. R., Jamnik, V. K., Bredin, S. S. D., McKenzie, D. C., Stone, J., Shephard, R. J. & Gledhill, N. (2011). 'Evidence-based risk assessment and recommendations for physical activity clearance: An introduction.' *Applied Physiology, Nutrition, and Metabolism*, 36(1), S1–2. https://doi.org/10.1139/h11-060

- Joy, E. A. & Pescatello, L. S. (2016). 'Pre-exercise screening: role of the primary care physician.' *Israel Journal of Health Policy Research*, 5, 29. https://doi.org/10.1186/s13584-016-0089-0

- Warburton, D. E. R., Jamnik, V. K., Bredin, S. S. D. & Gledhill, N. on behalf of the PAR-Q+ Collaboration. 'The Physical Activity Readiness Questionnaire for Everyone (PAR-Q+) and Electronic Physical Activity Readiness Medical Examination (ePARmed-X+).' *Health & Fitness Journal of Canada* 4(2):3-23, 2011. Available at: https://eparmedx.com/wp-content/uploads/2022/01/ParQPlus2022.pdf
- Simpson, R. J. & Katsanis, E. (2020). 'The immunological case for staying active during the COVID-19 pandemic.' *Brain, Behavior, and Immunity*, 87, 6–7. https://doi.org/10.1016/j.bbi.2020.04.041
- The Royal Australian College of General Practitioners. (2020). 'Returning to physical activity post-SARS-CoV-2 infection.' *Australian Journal of General Practice*, 49(11), Editorial. Available at: https://www1.racgp.org.au/getmedia/28358456-d646-4e74-a701-95012564332f/AJGP-11-2020-Editorial-Jewson-Life-After-COVID-19-Figure-1.pdf.aspx
- Bateman, L., Bested, A. C., Bonilla, H. F., Ruhoy, I. S., Vera-Nunez, M. A. & Yellman, B. P. (2021). 'Myalgic Encephalomyelitis/Chronic Fatigue Syndrome: Essentials of Diagnosis and Management.' *Mayo Clinic Proceedings*, 96(11), 2861–78. https://doi.org/10.1016/j.mayocp.2021.07.004
- World Health Organization. (2023, August 18). Clinical management of COVID-19: Living guideline. COVID-19: Clinical care. Available at: https://www.who.int/publications/i/item/WHO-2019-nCoV-clinical-2023.2
- Agency for Clinical Intervention (2022, July 15). 'COVID-19 Critical Intelligence Unit: Exercise and long COVID.' Available at: https://aci.health.nsw.gov.au/__data/assets/pdf_file/0010/735562/Evidence-Check-Exercise-and-long-COVID.pdf

- World Physiotherapy (2021). 'World Physiotherapy Response to COVID-19 Briefing Paper 9. Safe rehabilitation approaches for people living with Long COVID: physical activity and exercise.' London, UK: World Physiotherapy. ISBN: 978-1-914952-00-5. Available at: https://world.physio/sites/default/files/2021-07/Briefing-Paper-9-Long-Covid-FINAL-English-2021_0.pdf

Chapter 6: How to exercise with autoimmune conditions

- Ekkekakis, P. (2010). 'Pleasure and displeasure from the body: Perspectives from exercise.' *Journal of Sport and Exercise Psychology*, 25(2), 213–39. https://doi.org/10.1080/02699930302292
- Raedeke, T. D. (2007). 'The Relationship Between Enjoyment and Affective Responses to Exercise.' *Journal of Applied Sport Psychology*, 19(1), 105–15. https://doi.org/10.1080/10413200601113638
- Physical Activity Guidelines Advisory Committee (2008). 'Physical Activity Guidelines Advisory Committee Report, 2008.' Washington, DC: U.S. Department of Health and Human Services. https://health.gov/sites/default/files/2019-10/CommitteeReport_7.pdf
- Ries, A. L. (2005). 'Minimally Clinically Important Difference for the UCSD Shortness of Breath Questionnaire, Borg Scale, and Visual Analog Scale.' *COPD: Journal of Chronic Obstructive Pulmonary Disease*, 2(1), 105–10. https://doi.org/10.1081/COPD-200050655
- Riebe, D., Ehrman, J. K., Liguori, G. & Magal, M. (2018). 'General Principles of Exercise Prescription.' In ACSM's *Guidelines for Exercise Testing and Prescription* (10th ed., pp.

143–79). Wolters Kluwer/Lippincott Williams & Wilkins, Philadelphia, PA.

- Morishita, S., Tsubaki, A., Takabayashi, T. & Fu, J. B. (2018). 'Relationship between the rating of perceived exertion scale and the load intensity of resistance training.' *Strength and Conditioning Journal*, 40(2), 94–109. https://doi.org/10.1519/SSC.0000000000000373
- Borg, G. (1998). 'Borg's perceived exertion and pain scales.' *Human Kinetics.*
- Borg G. (1970). 'Perceived exertion as an indicator of somatic stress.' *Scandinavian Journal of Rehabilitation Medicine*, 2(2), 92–8. https://pubmed.ncbi.nlm.nih.gov/5523831/
- Chen, M. J., Fan, X. & Moe, S. T. (2002). 'Criterion-related validity of the Borg ratings of perceived exertion scale in healthy individuals: A meta-analysis.' *Journal of Sports Sciences*, 20(11), 873–99. https://doi.org/10.1080/026404102320761787

Chapter 7: Types of exercise

- World Health Organization (2022, October 5). 'Physical activity.' Available at: https://www.who.int/news-room/fact-sheets/detail/physical-activity
- Momma, H., Kawakami, R., Honda, T., et al. (2022). 'Muscle-strengthening activities are associated with lower risk and mortality in major non-communicable diseases: A systematic review and meta-analysis of cohort studies.' *British Journal of Sports Medicine*, 56, 755–63. https://doi.org/10.1136/bjsports-2021-105061
- Porter, S. & Wilson, J. (2020). *A Comprehensive Guide to Sports Physiology and Injury Management.* Elsevier. ISBN 978-0-7020-7489-9.

References

- Suchomel, T. J., Nimphius, S. & Stone, M. H. (2016). 'The Importance of Muscular Strength in Athletic Performance.' *Sports Medicine* (Auckland, N.Z.), 46(10), 1419–49. https://doi.org/10.1007/s40279-016-0486-0

- Bennie, J. A., Shakespear-Druery, J. & De Cocker, K. (2020). 'Muscle-strengthening Exercise Epidemiology: a New Frontier in Chronic Disease Prevention. *Sports Medicine – Open*, 6(1), 40. https://doi.org/10.1186/s40798-020-00271-w

- Garber, C. E., Blissmer, B., Deschenes, M. R., Franklin, B. A., Lamonte, M. J., Lee, I. M., Nieman, D. C., Swain, D. P. & American College of Sports Medicine (2011). 'Quantity and quality of exercise for developing and maintaining cardiorespiratory, musculoskeletal, and neuromotor fitness in apparently healthy adults: guidance for prescribing exercise.' *Medicine and Science in Sports and Exercise*, 43(7), 1334–59. https://doi.org/10.1249/MSS.0b013e318213fefb

- Ashton, R. E., Tew, G. A., Aning, J. J., Gilbert, S. E., Lewis, L. & Saxton, J. M. (2020). 'Effects of short-term, medium-term and long-term resistance exercise training on cardiometabolic health outcomes in adults: systematic review with meta-analysis. *British Journal of Sports medicine*, 54(6), 341–8. https://doi.org/10.1136/bjsports-2017-098970

- Mendes Sieczkowska, S., Reis Coimbra, D., Torres Vilarino, G., Andrade, A. (2020). 'Effects of resistance training on the health-related quality of life of patients with rheumatic diseases: Systematic review with meta-analysis and meta-regression.' *Seminars in Arthritis and Rheumatism*, 50(2), 342–53. https://doi.org/10.1016/j.semarthrit.2019.09.006.

- Yorks, D. M., Frothingham, C. A. & Schuenke, M. D. (2017). 'Effects of Group Fitness Classes on Stress and Quality of Life of Medical Students'. *Journal of Osteopathic Medicine*. Open

Access Published by De Gruyter. https://doi.org/10.7556/jaoa.2017.140

- Calık, B. B., Kabul, E. G., Korkmaz, C., Tekin, Z. E., Yener, G. O. & Yuksel, S. (2020). 'The efficacy of clinical Pilates exercises in children and adolescents with juvenile idiopathic arthritis: A pilot study.' *Revista Colombiana de Reumatología*, 27(4), 269–77. https://doi.org/10.1016/j.rcreu.2020.06.015

- Al-Qubaeissy, K. Y., Fatoye, F. A., Goodwin, P. C. & Yohannes, A. M. (2013). 'The effectiveness of hydrotherapy in the management of rheumatoid arthritis: a systematic review.' *Musculoskeletal Care*, 11(1), 3–18. https://doi.org/10.1002/msc.1028

- Markotić, V., Pokrajčić, V., Babić, M., Radančević, D., Grle, M., Miljko, M., Kosović, V., Jurić, I. & Karlović Vidaković, M. (2020). 'The Positive Effects of Running on Mental Health.' *Psychiatria Danubina*, 32(Suppl 2), 233–5. Available at: https://pubmed.ncbi.nlm.nih.gov/32970641/

- Oswald, F., Campbell, J., Williamson, C., Richards, J. & Kelly, P. (2020). 'A Scoping Review of the Relationship between Running and Mental Health.' *International Journal of Environmental Research and Public Health*, 17(21), 8059. https://doi.org/10.3390/ijerph17218059

- Lee, D.-c., Brellenthin, A. G., Thompson, P. D., Sui, X., Lee, I.-M. & Lavie, C. J. (2017). Running as a key lifestyle medicine for longevity.' *Progress in Cardiovascular Diseases*, 60(1), 45–55. https://doi.org/10.1016/j.pcad.2017.03.005

- Wen, C. P., Wai, J. P. M., Tsai, M. K., Chen, C. H. & Chen, M. K. (2014). 'Minimal Amount of Exercise to Prolong Life: To Walk, to Run, or Just Mix It Up?' *Journal of the American College of Cardiology*, 64(5), 482–4. https://doi.org/10.1016/j.jacc.2014.05.026

References

- Paty J. G., Jr (1994). 'Running injuries.' *Current Opinion in Rheumatology*, 6(2), 203–9. https://doi.org/10.1097/00002281-199403000-00015

- Massey, H., Gorczynski, P., Harper, C. M., Sansom, L., McEwan, K., Yankouskaya, A. & Denton, H. (2022). 'Perceived Impact of Outdoor Swimming on Health: Web-Based Survey.' *Interactive Journal of Medical Research*, 11(1), e25589. https://doi.org/10.2196/25589

- Shi, Z., Zhou, H., Lu, L., Pan, B., Wei, Z., Yao, X., Kang, Y., Liu, L. & Feng, S. (2018). 'Aquatic Exercises in the Treatment of Low Back Pain: A Systematic Review of the Literature and Meta-Analysis of Eight Studies.' *American Journal of Physical Medicine & Rehabilitation*, 97(2), 116–22. https://doi.org/10.1097/PHM.0000000000000801

- Ariyoshi, M., Sonoda, K., Nagata, K., Mashima, T., Zenmyo, M., Paku, C., Takamiya, Y., Yoshimatsu, H., Hirai, Y., Yasunaga, H., Akashi, H., Imayama, H., Shimokobe, T., Inoue, A. & Mutoh, Y. (1999). 'Efficacy of aquatic exercises for patients with low-back pain.' *The Kurume Medical Journal*, 46(2), 91–6. https://doi.org/10.2739/kurumemedj.46.91

- Jackson, M., Kang, M., Furness, J. & Kemp-Smith, K. (2022). 'Aquatic exercise and mental health: A scoping review.' *Complementary Therapies in Medicine*, 66, 102820. https://doi.org/10.1016/j.ctim.2022.102820

- Barker, A. L., Talevski, J., Morello, R. T., Brand, C. A., Rahmann, A. E. & Urquhart, D. M. (2014). 'Effectiveness of aquatic exercise for musculoskeletal conditions: a meta-analysis.' *Archives of Physical Medicine and Rehabilitation*, 95(9), 1776–86. https://doi.org/10.1016/j.apmr.2014.04.005

- Dundar, U., Solak, O., Toktas, H., Demirdal, U. S., Subasi, V., Kavuncu, V. & Evcik, D. (2014). 'Effect of aquatic exercise on ankylosing spondylitis: a randomized controlled trial.' *Rheumatology International*, 34(11), 1505–11. https://doi.org/10.1007/s00296-014-2980-8

- Zão, A., & Cantista, P. (2017). 'The role of land and aquatic exercise in ankylosing spondylitis: a systematic review.' *Rheumatology International*, 37(12), 1979–90. https://doi.org/10.1007/s00296-017-3829-8

- Medrado, L. N., Mendonça, M. L. M., Budib, M. B., Oliveira-Junior, S. A. & Martinez, P. F. (2022). 'Effectiveness of aquatic exercise in the treatment of inflammatory arthritis: systematic review.' *Rheumatology International*, 42(10), 1681–91. https://doi.org/10.1007/s00296-022-05145-w

- Al-Qubaeissy, K. Y., Fatoye, F. A., Goodwin, P. C. & Yohannes, A. M. (2013). 'The effectiveness of hydrotherapy in the management of rheumatoid arthritis: a systematic review.' *Musculoskeletal Care*, 11(1), 3–18. https://doi.org/10.1002/msc.1028

- Chen, M. H., DeLuca, J., Sandroff, B. M. & Genova, H. M. (2022). 'Aquatic exercise for persons with MS: Patient-reported preferences, obstacles and recommendations.' *Multiple Sclerosis and Related Disorders*, 60, 103701. https://doi.org/10.1016/j.msard.2022.103701

- So, B. C. L., Kwok, S. C. & Lee, P. H. (2021). 'Effect of Aquatic Exercise on Sleep Efficiency of Adults With Chronic Musculoskeletal Pain.' *Journal of Physical Activity and Health*, 18(9), 1037–45. https://doi.org/10.1123/jpah.2020-0476

- Paluch, A. E., Gabriel, K. P., Fulton, J. E., et al. (2021). 'Steps per Day and All-Cause Mortality in Middle-aged Adults in the Coronary Artery Risk Development in Young Adults Study.' *JAMA Network Open*, 4(9), e2124516. https://doi.org/10.1001/jamanetworkopen.2021.24516

References

- Dwyer, T., Pezic, A., Sun, C., Cochrane, J., Venn, A., Srikanth, V., Jones, G., Shook, R., Sui, X., Ortaglia, A., Blair, S. & Ponsonby, L. (2015). 'Objectively Measured Daily Steps and Subsequent Long Term All-Cause Mortality: The Tasped Prospective Cohort Study.' *PLOS One*, 10(11), e0141274. https://doi.org/10.1371/journal.pone.0141274

- Peñacoba, C., Pastor, M. Á., López-Roig, S., Velasco, L. & Lledo, A. (2017). 'Walking Beliefs in Women With Fibromyalgia: Clinical Profile and Impact on Walking Behavior.' *Clinical Nursing Research*, 26(5), 632–50. https://doi.org/10.1177/1054773816646339

- Omura, J. D., Ussery, E. N., Loustalot, F., Fulton, J. E. & Carlson, S. A. (2019). 'Walking as an Opportunity for Cardiovascular Disease Prevention.' *Preventing Chronic Disease*, 16, E66. https://doi.org/10.5888/pcd16.180690

- Mau, M., Aaby, A., Klausen, S. H. & Roessler, K. K. (2021). 'Are Long-Distance Walks Therapeutic? A Systematic Scoping Review of the Conceptualization of Long-Distance Walking and Its Relation to Mental Health.' *International Journal of Environmental Research and Public Health*, 18(15), 7741. https://doi.org/10.3390/ijerph18157741

- Kelly, P., Williamson, C., Niven, A. G., et al. (2018). 'Walking on sunshine: Scoping review of the evidence for walking and mental health.' *British Journal of Sports Medicine*, 52, 800–6. http://dx.doi.org/10.1136/bjsports-2017-098827

- Murtagh, E. M., Nichols, L., Mohammed, M. A., Holder, R., Nevill, A. M. & Murphy, M. H. (2015). 'The effect of walking on risk factors for cardiovascular disease: an updated systematic review and meta-analysis of randomised control trials.' *Preventive Medicine*, 72, 34–43. https://doi.org/10.1016/j.ypmed.2014.12.041

- O'Connor, S. R., Tully, M. A., Ryan, B., Bleakley, C. M., Baxter, G. D., Bradley, J. M. & McDonough, S. M. (2015). 'Walking Exercise for Chronic Musculoskeletal Pain: Systematic Review and Meta-Analysis.' *Archives of Physical Medicine and Rehabilitation*. Available at: https://core.ac.uk/reader/33583364?utm_source=linkout

- Hori, H., Ikenouchi-Sugita, A., Yoshimura, R., et al. (2016). 'Does subjective sleep quality improve by a walking intervention? A real-world study in a Japanese workplace.' *BMJ Open*, 6, e011055 https://bmjopen.bmj.com/content/6/10/e011055

- Tang, M. F., Chiu, H. Y., Xu, X., Kwok, J. Y., Cheung, D. S. T., Chen, C. Y. & Lin, C. C. (2019). 'Walking is more effective than yoga at reducing sleep disturbance in cancer patients: A systematic review and meta-analysis of randomized controlled trials.' *Sleep Medicine Reviews*, 47, 1–8. https://doi.org/10.1016/j.smrv.2019.05.003

- Celis-Morales, C. A., Gray, S., Petermann, F., Iliodromiti, S., Welsh, P., Lyall, D. M., Anderson, J., Pellicori, P., Mackay, D. F., Pell, J. P., Sattar, N. & Gill, J. M. R. (2019). 'Walking pace is associated with lower risk of all-cause and cause-specific mortality.' *Medicine & Science in Sports & Exercise*, 51(3), 472–80. https://doi.org/10.1249/MSS.0000000000001795

- Polaski, A. M., Phelps, A. L., Kostek, M. C., Szucs, K. A. & Kolber, B. J. (2019). 'Exercise-induced hypoalgesia: A meta-analysis of exercise dosing for the treatment of chronic pain.' *PlOS One*, 14(1), e0210418. https://doi.org/10.1371/journal.pone.0210418

- López-Roig, S., Ecija, C., Peñacoba, C., Ivorra, S., Nardi-Rodríguez, A., Lecuona, O. & Pastor-Mira, M. A. (2022).

References

'Assessing Walking Programs in Fibromyalgia: A Concordance Study between Measures.' *International Journal of Environmental Research and Public Health*, 19(5), 2995. https://doi.org/10.3390/ijerph19052995

- Woodyard C. (2011). 'Exploring the therapeutic effects of yoga and its ability to increase quality of life.' *International Journal of Yoga*, 4(2), 49–54. https://doi.org/10.4103/0973-6131.85485
- Cohen, L., Warneke, C., Fouladi, R. T., Rodriguez, M. A. & Chaoul-Reich, A. (2004). 'Psychological adjustment and sleep quality in a randomized trial of the effects of a Tibetan yoga intervention in patients with lymphoma.' *Cancer*, 100(10), 2253–60. https://doi.org/10.1002/cncr.20236
- Pilkington, K., Kirkwood, G., Rampes, H. & Richardson, J. (2005). 'Yoga for depression: the research evidence.' *Journal of Affective Disorders*, 89(1–3), 13–24. https://doi.org/10.1016/j.jad.2005.08.013
- Gautam, S., Kumar, U., Kumar, M., Rana, D. & Dada, R. (2021). 'Yoga improves mitochondrial health and reduces severity of autoimmune inflammatory arthritis: A randomized controlled trial.' *Mitochondrion*, 58, 147–59. https://doi.org/10.1016/j.mito.2021.03.004
- Rogers, K. A. & MacDonald, M. (2015). 'Therapeutic Yoga: Symptom Management for Multiple Sclerosis.' *The Journal of Alternative and Complementary Medicine* (New York, N.Y.), 21(11), 655–9. https://doi.org/10.1089/acm.2015.0015
- Fargo, M. & Wilkins, B. (2023, March 28). '13 Types of Yoga Explained by the Experts + How to Pick the Right Style for You.' *Yoga Today*. https://www.womenshealthmag.com/uk/fitness/yoga/a25706715/types-of-yoga/

- Peng P. W. (2012). 'Tai chi and chronic pain.' *Regional anesthesia & Pain Medicine*, 37(4), 372–82. https://doi.org/10.1097/AAP.obo13e31824f6629

- Oh, B., Bae, K., Lamoury, G., Eade, T., Boyle, F., Corless, B., Clarke, S., Yeung, A., Rosenthal, D., Schapira, L. & Back, M. (2020). 'The Effects of Tai Chi and Qigong on Immune Responses: A Systematic Review and Meta-Analysis.' *Medicines* (Basel, Switzerland), 7(7), 39. https://doi.org/10.3390/medicines7070039

- Jahnke, R., Larkey, L., Rogers, C., Etnier, J. & Lin, F. (2010). 'A comprehensive review of health benefits of qigong and tai chi.' *American Journal of Health Promotion (AJHP)*, 24(6), e1–e25. https://doi.org/10.4278/ajhp.081013-LIT-248

- Litscher, G., Zhang, W., Huang, T. & Wang, L. (2011). 'Heart rate and heart rate variability responses to Tai Chi and jogging in Beijing and Graz.' *North American Journal of Medical Sciences*, 3(2), 70–4. https://doi.org/10.4297/najms.2011.370

Chapter 10: Adapting exercise

- Hellström, B., & Anderberg, U. M. (2003). 'Pain perception across the menstrual cycle phases in women with chronic pain.' *Perceptual and Motor Skills*, 96(1), 201–11. https://doi.org/10.2466/pms.2003.96.1.201

- Tan, B., Philipp, M., Hill, S., Che Muhamed, A. M. & Mündel, T. (2020). 'Pain Across the Menstrual Cycle: Considerations of Hydration.' *Frontiers in Physiology*, 11, 585667. https://doi.org/10.3389/fphys.2020.585667

- Kozinoga, M., Majchrzycki, M. & Piotrowska, S. (2015). 'Low back pain in women before and after menopause'. *Przeglad menopauzalny/Menopause Review*, 14(3), 203–7. https://doi. org/10.5114/pm.2015.54347

- Zelaya, C. E., Dahlhamer, J. M., Lucas, J. W. & Connor, E. M. (2020). 'Chronic pain and high-impact chronic pain among U.S. adults, 2019.' NCHS Data Brief, No. 390. Hyattsville, MD: National Center for Health Statistics. Available at: https://www.cdc.gov/nchs/data/databriefs/db390-H.pdf

- Gibson, C. J., Li, Y., Bertenthal, D., Huang, A. J. Seal, K. H. (2019). 'Menopause symptoms and chronic pain in a national sample of midlife women veterans.' *Menopause*, 26(7), 708–13. https://doi.org/10.1097/GME.0000000000001312

- American College of Sports Medicine (2011). 'Delayed onset muscle soreness.' Copyright © 2011 American College of Sports Medicine. Created and updated by William Braun, Ph.D., and Gary Sforzo, Ph.D. Product of ACSM's Consumer Information Committee. Available at: https://www.acsm.org/docs/default-source/files-for-resource-library/delayed-onset-muscle-soreness-%28doms%29.pdf

- Peake, J. M., Neubauer, O., Della Gatta, P. A. & Nosaka, K. (2017). 'Muscle damage and inflammation during recovery from exercise.' *Journal of Applied Physiology*, 122(3), 559–70. https://doi.org/10.1152/japplphysiol.00971.2016

- Sports Science for Coaches (25 January 2015). 'Exercise Induced Muscle Damage.' Available from: https://sportsscienceforcoaches. wordpress.com/2015/01/25/exercise-induced-muscle-damage/

- Toumi, H. & Best, T. M. (2003). 'The inflammatory response: friend or enemy for muscle injury?' *British Journal of Sports Medicine*, 37(4), 284–286. https://doi.org/10.1136/bjsm.37.4.284

- Macciochi, J. (2022). *Your Blueprint for Strong Immunity: Personalise Your Diet and Lifestyle for Better Health*. Yellow Kite.

- Wallace, H. (2022). *The Female Factor: Making Women's Health Count and What It Means for You*. Yellow Kite.
- Dettmer, P. (2021). *Immune: A Journey into the Mysterious System That Keeps You Alive*. Hodder & Stoughton.

Chapter 11: Exercising with fatigue

- Riley, W. T., Rothrock, N., Bruce, B., Christodolou, C., Cook, K., Hahn, E. A. & Cella, D. (2010). 'Patient-reported outcomes measurement information system (PROMIS) domain names and definitions revisions: further evaluation of content validity in IRT-derived item banks.' *Quality of Life Research*, 19(9), 1311–21. https://doi.org/10.1007/s11136-010-9694-5
- Miserandino, C. (n.d.). 'The Spoon Theory'.
- Dalton-Smith, S. D. (n.d.). *Sacred Rest: Recover Your Life, Renew Your Energy, Restore Your Sanity*. FaithWords.
- Mograss, M., Abi-Jaoude, J., Frimpong, E., Chalati, D., Moretto, U., Tarelli, L., Lim, A. & Dang-Vu, T. T. (2022). 'The effects of napping on night-time sleep in healthy young adults.' *Journal of Sleep Research*, 31(3), e13578. https://doi.org/10.1111/jsr.13578
- Milner, C. E. & Cote, K. A. (2009). 'Benefits of napping in healthy adults: Impact of nap length, time of day, age, and experience with napping.' *Journal of Sleep Research*, 18(2), 272-281. https://doi.org/10.1111/j.1365-2869.2008.00718.x
- Goldschmied, J. R., Cheng, P., Kemp, K., Caccamo, L., Roberts, J. & Deldin, P. J. (2015). 'Napping to modulate frustration and impulsivity: A pilot study.' *Personality and Individual Differences*, 86, 164–7. https://doi.org/10.1016/j.paid.2015.06.013
- Weir, K. (2016). 'The science of naps: Researchers are working to pinpoint the benefits — and possible drawbacks — of an

afternoon snooze.' *Monitor on Psychology*, 47(7), 48. Available at: https://www.apa.org/monitor/2016/07-08/naps

- Mednick, S., Nakayama, K. & Stickgold, R. (2003). 'Sleep-dependent learning: A nap is as good as a night.' *Nature Neuroscience*, 6(7), 697–8. https://doi.org/10.1038/nn1078
- Dautovich, N. D., McCrae, C. S. & Rowe, M. (2008). 'Subjective and Objective Napping and Sleep in Older Adults: Are Evening Naps "Bad" for Nighttime Sleep?' *Journal of the American Geriatrics Society*, 56(9), 1681–6. https://doi.org/10.1111/j.1532-5415.2008.01822.x
- Shoji, K. D., Tighe, C. A., Imel, J. L., Dautovich, N. D. & McCrae, C. M. (2016). 'Napping in Older and College-Aged Adults.' *Journal of the American Geriatrics Society*, 64(4), 896–8. https://doi.org/10.1111/jgs.14056
- Gotts, Z. M., Ellis, J. G., Deary, V., Barclay, N. & Newton, J. L. (2015). 'The Association between Daytime Napping and Cognitive Functioning in Chronic Fatigue Syndrome.' *PLOS One*, 10(1), e0117136. https://doi.org/10.1371/journal.pone.0117136
- Jason, L., Benton, M., Torres-Harding, S. & Muldowney, K. (2009). 'The impact of energy modulation on physical functioning and fatigue severity among patients with ME/CFS.' *Patient Education and Counseling*, 77(2), 237–41. https://doi.org/10.1016/j.pec.2009.02.015
- Jason, L., Muldowney, K. & Torres-Harding, S. (2008). 'The Energy Envelope Theory and myalgic encephalomyelitis/chronic fatigue syndrome.' *AAOHN Journal: Official Journal of the American Association of Occupational Health Nurses*, 56(5), 189–95. https://doi.org/10.3928/08910162-20080501-06

- Van Campen, C., Rowe, P. & Visser, F. (2020). 'Heart Rate Thresholds to Limit Activity in Myalgic Encephalomyelitis/ Chronic Fatigue Syndrome Patients (Pacing): Comparison of Heart Rate Formulae and Measurements of the Heart Rate at the Lactic Acidosis Threshold during Cardiopulmonary Exercise Testing.' *Advances in Physical Education*, 10(2), 138–54. https://doi.org/10.4236/ape.2020.102013
- Boissoneault, J., Letzen, J., Robinson, M. & Staud, R. (2019). 'Cerebral blood flow and heart rate variability predict fatigue severity in patients with chronic fatigue syndrome.' *Brain Imaging and Behavior*, 13(3), 789–7. https://doi.org/10.1007/s11682-018-9897-x
- Ni, Z., Sun, F. & Li, Y. (2022). 'Heart Rate Variability-Based Subjective Physical Fatigue Assessment.' *Sensors* (Basel, Switzerland), 22(9), 3199. https://doi.org/10.3390/s22093199
- Wasserman K. (1986). 'The anaerobic threshold: definition, physiological significance and identification.' *Advances in Cardiology*, 35, 1–23. Available at: https://europepmc.org/article/med/3551513
- Cornelissen, V., Verheyden, B., Aubert, A., et al. (2010). 'Effects of aerobic training intensity on resting, exercise and post-exercise blood pressure, heart rate and heart-rate variability.' *Journal of Human Hypertension*, 24(3), 175–82. https://doi.org/10.1038/jhh.2009.51

Chapter 12: Exercising with pain

- Butler, D. & Moseley, L. (2015). *Explain Pain*. Noigroup Publications.

- Moseley, G. L. & Butler, D. S. (2022). *The Explain Pain Handbook: Protectometer*. NOI Group Publications.

- Marchand, F., Perretti, M. & McMahon, S. (2005). 'Role of the immune system in chronic pain.' *Nature Reviews Neuroscience*, 6, 521–32. https://doi.org/10.1038/nrn1700.

- Jensen, M. P., Turner, J. A., Romano, J. M. & Karoly, P. (1991). 'Coping with chronic pain: A critical review of the literature.' *Pain*, 47(3), 249–83. https://doi.org/10.1016/0304-3959(91)90216-K.

- Lamé, I. E., Peters, M. L., Vlaeyen, J. W. S., v. Kleef, M. & Patijn, J. (2005). 'Quality of life in chronic pain is more associated with beliefs about pain than with pain intensity.' *European Journal of Pain*, 9(1), 15–24. https://doi.org/10.1016/j.ejpain.2004.02.006

- Breit, S., Kupferberg, A., Rogler, G. & Hasler, G. (2018). 'Vagus Nerve as Modulator of the Brain-Gut Axis in Psychiatric and Inflammatory Disorders.' *Frontiers in Psychiatry*, 9, 44. https://doi.org/10.3389/fpsyt.2018.00044

- Frangos, E., Richards, E. A. & Bushnell, M. C. (2017). 'Do the psychological effects of vagus nerve stimulation partially mediate vagal pain modulation?' *Neurobiology of Pain*, 1, 37–45. https://doi.org/10.1016/j.ynpai.2017.03.002

Chapter 13: Mindset and movement

- Torrijos-Zarcero, M., Mediavilla, R., Rodríguez-Vega, B., Del Río-Diéguez, M., López-Álvarez, I., Rocamora-González, C. & Palao-Tarrero, Á. (2021). 'Mindful Self-Compassion program for chronic pain patients: A randomized controlled trial.' *European Journal of Pain* (London, England), 25(4), 930–44. https://doi.org/10.1002/ejp.1734

- Kılıç, A., Hudson, J., McCracken, L. M., Ruparelia, R., Fawson, S. & Hughes, L. D. (2021). 'A Systematic Review of the Effectiveness of Self-Compassion-Related Interventions for Individuals With Chronic Physical Health Conditions.' *Behavior Therapy*, 52(3), 607–25. https://doi.org/10.1016/j.beth.2020.08.001

Index

Acknowledgements

Thank you, Carolyn Thorne, for believing in me from the start; despite my initial doubts that I could write a book, you made it happen. Thanks for your guidance, accommodating my unpredictable health and being kind every step of the way. Emily Johnson, your offer to contribute to your book opened the door to mine, so thank you for asking me. Big thanks to the talented artist, Wioleta Deptula, and to the editors and team at Yellow Kite who shaped this book so brilliantly, making me, a newbie, become an author.

My husband, Dejan, your love, humour and support have been crucial amid the chaos of our busy year. To my parents, thank you for everything. Especially Mum, for deciphering early drafts and supporting me through daily video calls, and to Dad, Rory and Helen, thanks for always being my biggest fans whatever I do. Dragan, Lidija, Ali and Sasha, thanks for being my official family now.

Chloe, Ellie and Laura, thanks for always being there, no matter the distance. To the Girl Gang – Nat, Soph, Evie, Amy and Carolyn – your virtual support during my tough times with chronic illness means the world. Michelle, thanks for always being right there (literally).

To my medical team – especially Dr Ginges, Dr Dally, Prof Carmody, Prof Spiros and Tim Oxbrow – thanks for helping my

Acknowledgements

body to function over the years. John Larner, David Schofield, Lucia Berry and Lana Johnson, thank you for shaping me into the physio-therapist I am today. Melissa Williams, your Physio approval gave me the confidence to share this book, thanks for your wisdom.

To all my clients, thanks for trusting me to be part of your journey and letting me learn alongside you. And to everyone who follows my journey on Actively Autoimmune, your support has been incredible and none of this would have happened without it. I am so grateful for each one of you.

About the author

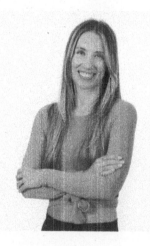

Zoe Mckenzie is founder of the online platform activelyautoimmune.com. She is a qualified physiotherapist, PT and Pilates instructor specialising in helping people who suffer with autoimmune conditions. After an early diagnosis of Ehlers Danlos Type III, she progressed from using a wheelchair to learning how to walk again. She has had 20 years' experience of living with multiple chronic conditions. She uses exercise as a daily management tool and wants to inspire, educate and support the invisible illness community.

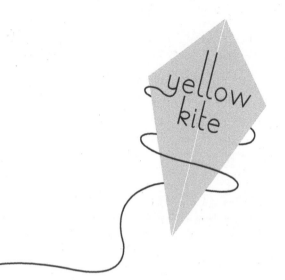

books to help you live a good life

Join the conversation and tell
us how you live a #goodlife

🐦 @yellowkitebooks
f YellowKiteBooks
📌 Yellow Kite Books
📷 YellowKiteBooks